Sexual Health

Understanding Public Health Series

Series editors: Nicki Thorogood and Ros Plowman, London School of Hygiene & Tropical Medicine (previous edition edited by Nick Black and Rosalind Raine)

Throughout the world, there is growing recognition of the importance of public health to sustainable, safe, and healthy societies. The achievements of public health in nineteenth-century Europe were for much of the twentieth century overshadowed by advances in personal care, in particular in hospital care. Now, with the dawning of a new century, there is increasing understanding of the inevitable limits of individual health care and of the need to complement such services with effective public health strategies. Major improvements in people's health will come from controlling communicable diseases, eradicating environmental hazards, improving people's diets, and enhancing the availability and quality of effective health care. To achieve this, every country needs a cadre of knowledgeable public health practitioners with social, political, and organizational skills to lead and bring about changes at international, national, and local levels.

This is one of a series of books that provides a foundation for those wishing to join in and contribute to the twenty-first-century regeneration of public health, helping to put the concerns and perspectives of public health at the heart of policy-making and service provision. While each book stands alone, together they provide a comprehensive account of the three main aims of public health: protecting the public from environmental hazards, improving the health of the public, and ensuring high-quality health services are available to all. Some of the books focus on methods, others on key topics. They have been written by staff at the London School of Hygiene & Tropical Medicine with considerable experience of teaching public health to students from low-, middle-, and high-income countries. Much of the material has been developed and tested with postgraduate students both in face-to-face teaching and through distance learning.

The books are designed for self-directed learning. Each chapter has explicit learning objectives, key terms are highlighted, and the text contains many activities to enable the reader to test their own understanding of the ideas and material covered. Written in a clear and accessible style, the series will be essential reading for students taking postgraduate courses in public health and will also be of interest to public health practitioners and policy-makers.

Titles in the series

Analytical models for decision making: Colin Sanderson and Reinhold Gruen
Conflict and health: Natasha Howard, Egbert Sondorp and Annemarie ter Veen (eds.)
Controlling communicable disease: Norman Noah
Economic analysis for management and policy: Stephen Jan, Lilani Kumaranayake, Jenny Roberts, Kara Hanson and Kate Archibald
Economic evaluation: Julia Fox-Rushby and John Cairns (eds.)
Environmental epidemiology: Paul Wilkinson (ed.)
Environmental health policy: Megan Landon and Tony Fletcher
Financial management in health services: Reinhold Gruen and Anne Howarth
Global change and health: Kelley Lee and Jeff Collin (eds.)
Health care evaluation: Sarah Smith, Don Sinclair, Rosalind Raine and Barnaby Reeves
Health promotion practice: Maggie Davies, Wendy Macdowall and Chris Bonell (eds.)
Health promotion theory: Maggie Davies and Wendy Macdowall (eds.)
Introduction to epidemiology, Second Edition: Ilona Carneiro and Natasha Howard
Introduction to health economics, Second Edition: Lorna Guinness and Virginia Wiseman (eds.)
Issues in public health, Second Edition: Fiona Sim and Martin McKee (eds.)
Making health policy, Second Edition: Kent Buse, Nicholas Mays and Gill Walt
Managing health services: Nick Goodwin, Reinhold Gruen and Valerie Iles
Medical anthropology: Robert Pool and Wenzel Geissler
Principles of social research: Judith Green and John Browne (eds.)
Public health in history: Virginia Berridge, Martin Gorsky and Alex Mold
Sexual health: a public health perspective: Kaye Wellings, Kirstin Mitchell and Martine Collumbien (eds.)
Understanding health services: Nick Black and Reinhold Gruen

Forthcoming titles

Environment, health and sustainable development, Second Edition: Sari Kovats and Emma Hutchinson (eds.)

Sexual Health

A public health perspective

Edited by Kaye Wellings, Kirstin Mitchell
and Martine Collumbien

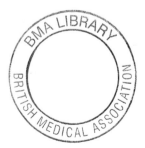

Open University Press

Open University Press
McGraw-Hill Education
McGraw-Hill House
Shoppenhangers Road
Maidenhead
Berkshire
England
SL6 2QL

email: enquiries@openup.co.uk
world wide web: www.openup.co.uk

and Two Penn Plaza, New York, NY 10121-2289, USA

First published 2012

A catalogue record of this book is available from the British Library

ISBN-13: 978-0-33-524481-2 (pb)
ISBN-10: 0-33-524481-5 (pb)
eISBN: 978-0-33-524482-9

Library of Congress Cataloging-in-Publication Data
CIP data applied for

Typesetting and e-book compilations by
RefineCatch Limited, Bungay, Suffolk
Printed in the UK by Bell & Bain Ltd, Glasgow

Fictitious names of companies, products, people, characters and/or data that may be used
herein (in case studies or in examples) are not intended to represent any real individual,
company, product or event.

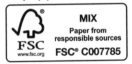

MIX
Paper from
responsible sources
FSC® C007785

Contents

List of figures, tables and boxes

Figures

Tables

Boxes

Preface

In writing this book, we have invited contributions from a variety of specialists in the field of sexual health, and inevitably, each has their own perspectives, preferences and priorities. One unifying theme runs throughout the book however, and that is the importance of social context in shaping not only sexual health status, but also efforts to improve it.

In the first section of the book, we chart some of the many perspectives guiding the study of sexual health, and we identify those we believe to be most valuably applied in a public health context. Section 2 includes four chapters representing key areas of sexual health which form the endpoints for public health intervention designed to improve sexual health status: sexually transmitted infection, unplanned pregnancy, sexual violence and sexual function. In doing so we adopt a broad definition of sexual health – one which emphasizes not only biomedical goals relating to fertility and infection, but also behavioural ones which encompasses not only negative but also positive aspects of sexual health, such as well-being and satisfaction.

In section 3 we identify the different foci of these efforts, in terms of risk and audience groups, and also the social context. In section 4, we explore ways in which public health endeavours operate to improve sexual health status: by communicating clearly, by providing appropriate sex education and health services, and by adopting preventive strategies. Finally, in section 5, we examine the roles of research and evaluation in informing intervention design and in assessing progress towards the goal of improving sexual health status.

Acknowledgements

The editors would like to thank Adam Fletcher, Ros Plowman, and Nicki Thorogood for their helpful comments on the manuscript. We are also grateful to Rachael Parker for her patient administrative support. The greatest debt is to LSHTM Masters students who, during successive years of taking the Sexual Health course, have helped shape the editors' understanding of sexual health and provided a wealth of illustrations from their own experience.

Open University Press and the London School of Hygiene & Tropical Medicine have made every effort to obtain permission from copyright holders to reproduce material in this book and to acknowledge these sources correctly. Any omissions brought to our attention will be remedied in future editions.

We would like to express our grateful thanks to the copyright holders for granting permission to reproduce material in this book from the following sources:

Bancroft J (2009) *Human Sexuality and its Problems*. London: Elsevier. By permission of Elsevier Press.

Copas A, Wellings K, Erens B, Mercer CH, McManus S, Fenton KA, Macdowall W, Nanchahal K and Johnson AM (2002) The accuracy of reported sensitive sexual behaviour in Britain: exploring the extent of change 1990–2000, *Sexually Transmitted Infections*, 78(1): 26–30. By permission of the BMJ Publishing Group Ltd.

Sandfort TGM and Ehrhardt AA (2004) Sexual health: a useful public health paradigm or a moral imperative?, *Archives of Sexual Behaviour*, 33(3): 181–7. By permission of Oxford University Press.

Slaymaker E, Bwanika JB, Kasamba I, Lutalo T, Maher D and Todd J (2009) Trends in age at first sex in Uganda: evidence from demographic and health survey data and longitudinal cohorts in Masaka and Rakai, *Sexually Transmitted Infections*, 85(supp.11): i12–i19. By permission of Emma Slaymaker.

Trussell J (2011) Contraceptive efficacy, in RA Hatcher, J Trussell, AL Nelson, W Cates, D Kowal and M Policar (eds.) *Contraceptive Technology*, 20th revised edn. New York: Ardent Media. By permission of Deborah Kowal (Executive Editor of *Contraceptive Technology*) and James Trussell.

Wellings K, Collumbien M, Slaymaker E, Singh S, Hodges Z, Patel D and Bajos N (2006) Sexual behaviour in context: a global perspective, *Lancet*, 368(9548), 1706–28. By permission of Elsevier Press.

World Health Organization (1994) *ICD-10: International Statistical Classification of Diseases and Related Health Problems*, 10th edn. Geneva: WHO. By permission of the World Health Organization.

World Health Organization (2005) *WHO Multi-country Study on Women's Health and Domestic Violence against Women. Summary Report – Initial Results on Prevalence, Health Outcomes and Women's Responses.* Geneva: WHO. By permission of the World Health Organization.

PART I

Conceptual and theoretical aspects of sexual health

Sexual health: theoretical perspectives

Kaye Wellings

Overview

In this opening chapter, we introduce the perspectives that guide the book. We examine how sexual health might be defined and the criteria used to do so. We summarize the main theoretical approaches to sexuality, in particular the distinction between those that see it as relatively instinctual and fixed, and those that see it as socially learned and as capable of being modified. We make the case for adopting the second of these perspectives in the context of public health practice, and we emphasize the importance of taking account of the social and historical context in efforts to understand sexual health issues, thereby setting the scene for the whole book. Next, we introduce the concepts of diversity and normality and examine their application in the context of sexual behaviour. Finally, we consider some of the social and cultural constraints on sexual behaviour and how these impact on public health efforts to improve sexual health.

Learning outcomes

After reading this chapter, you will be able to:

- Critically appraise a definition of sexual health
- Identify different theoretical approaches to the study of sexual behaviour, and understand the arguments for applying a social learning model to public health practice
- Understand the importance of considering cultural and social factors shaping sexual behaviour and sexual health interventions

Key terms

Sex: In everyday speech, the term 'sex' is used to refer both to sexual activity (for example, 'having sex', 'sex work') and to the sum of biological characteristics that define people as female and male. In this book, we use the term in both these senses and rely on the context to make clear in which it is being used.

Sexuality: A core human dimension that includes sex, gender, sexual identity and orientation, eroticism, attachment and reproduction, and is experienced or expressed in thoughts, fantasies, desires, beliefs, attitudes, values, practices, roles, and relationships. Sexuality is a result of the interplay of biological, psychological, socio-economic, cultural, ethical, and religious/spiritual factors.

A public health approach

Throughout this book, we take a public health approach to sexual health, typified by the following characteristics:

- *The focus is on the health of populations, rather than on that of individuals.* The social patterning of, and trends in, sexual ill health are a key focus, as is a concern with reducing inequalities.
- *The emphasis is on prevention of ill health and promotion of wellbeing*, rather than on cure and treatment. Prevention may be primary, where the focus is on modifying behaviours that expose individuals to sexual ill health, for example, unprotected sexual intercourse; secondary, where incipient disease or risk behaviours are prevented from progressing, as in the case of screening for cervical cancer or provision of emergency contraception; or tertiary, where the impact of already established ill health is attenuated, as in the case of public education campaigns aimed at countering discrimination against people with HIV infection.
- Those designing public health interventions typically ask what factors can be most effectively modified to improve health status and these are seen to include not only behavioural factors determining individual risk, but also social structural factors impacting on the vulnerability of social groups or populations, (MacDougall, 2007) as discussed in Chapter 10.

Sexual health: an emerging concept

Despite its relatively recent origin (Sandfort and Erhardt, 2004), the term 'sexual health' is in increasingly common currency (Giami, 2002) (see Figure 1.1). This reflects a shift in public health thinking that has implications for both research and practice. Most

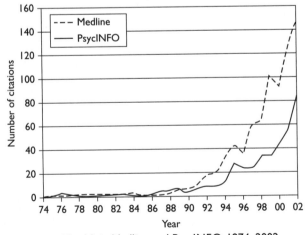

Figure 1.1 References to sexual health in Medline and PsycINFO, 1974–2002

notably, it marks a move away from the medicalization of the specialty. Formerly, labels attached to this area of public health practice carried connotations of disease and pathology. Settings in which sexual health care was practised, for example, tended to be named according to disease categories (for example, venereal disease clinic), or else were so euphemistically identified (as in 'special clinic') as to suggest something extraordinary or morally questionable. The trend away from medicalization is mirrored in research: empirical work is increasingly focused on behaviour rather than pathology; concerned with prevention as well as treatment; carried out by interdisciplinary teams of clinicians and social scientists, often combining laboratory and behavioural measures; and conducted in communities rather than clinics.

Defining sexual health

There is surprisingly little agreement on how the concept of sexual health should be defined. The most frequently cited definition was originally formulated at a conference held by the World Health Organization (WHO) in 1975, as a guide for health professionals working in the field. This definition went through several iterations. It was revised in a report in 2001 by a panel including the WHO, the Pan-American Health Organization (PAHO), and the World Association of Sexology (WAS) and further modified in 2002, when the WHO published a definition on the section of its website devoted to gender and reproductive rights.

> Sexual health is a state of physical, emotional, and social well-being in relation to sexuality; it is not merely the absence of disease, dysfunction or infirmity. Sexual health requires a positive and respectful approach to sexuality and sexual relationships, as well as the possibility of having pleasurable and safe sexual experiences, free of coercion, discrimination and violence. For sexual health to be attained and maintained, the sexual rights of all persons must be respected, protected and fulfilled.
>
> (WHO, 2006)

The WHO definition of sexual health has much to commend it. A holistic approach safeguards against seeing sexual health exclusively in terms of the prevention of adverse sexual health outcomes, such as unplanned pregnancy, sexually transmitted infections (STIs), and sexual violence. It expressly incorporates more positive aspects of sexual health, broadening the remit to include the enhancement of life and personal relations. Yet this definition has never been officially accepted in WHO terms of reference (even now, it is difficult to find on the WHO website). This may be because the inclusion of sexual satisfaction alongside adverse health outcomes makes some people uncomfortable. It may also reflect the inherent challenges associated with all 'positive' definitions of health (not just sexual health), particularly the vagueness of 'a state of physical, emotional and social well-being', the difficulty in anyone ever attaining this, and the challenges of measuring it. The WHO definition has, nevertheless, been used to help frame this book. The subjects of our opening chapters, the four most common outcomes in terms of interventions to improve sexual health – that is, unplanned pregnancy, sexually transmitted infection, sexual violence, and sexual function – correspond roughly to those incorporated in the WHO definition.

Theoretical perspectives

Broadly speaking, theories about sexuality fall into two main categories: the essentialist and the social constructionist (DeLamater and Hyde, 1998). *Essentialist* theories hold that forms of sexual expression are for the most part fixed, innate, and instinctual, that sex is determined chiefly by biological forces, even though situational and environmental factors may give rise to variation. *Social constructionist* theories, by contrast, regard sexual behaviour as plastic and malleable, amenable to modification, and shaped extensively by cultural norms and socialization, often mediated by language as a way of organizing experience and sharing concepts. While few hold the extreme view that either nature or nurture is totally responsible for determining human sexual behaviour, perspectives vary greatly in their relative emphasis. The task here is to examine each for its usefulness in a public health context.

Essentialist theories: sexuality as instinctual and innate

The belief that the determinants of sexual expression are to be found in instinct has a long history, dating from Plato and Aristotle, appearing in the Middle Ages in the concept of natural law (Weeks, 2003) and resurfacing in the writings of late nineteenth-century sexologists such as Krafft-Ebbing, Havelock Ellis, Magnus Hirschfeld, and Sigmund Freud. The fashionable view in this latter period was to see the study of sex as a science, observing natural laws. The aim was to uncover a single, timeless, incontrovertible truth about sexuality that could be discovered from, and had its origin in, biology and psychology. Chromosomes and hormones, and psychic energy or unconscious compulsions, were the building blocks of sexuality.

The concept of sex as a biological imperative was reflected in much of the language used by early sexologists. Freud, for example, describes sex as a 'drive' (Freud 1949) and Havelock Ellis as an 'impulse'. Implicit in the use of these terms is the notion of an uncontrollable natural energy in men and women (but particularly men) urgently seeking release. For Freud, the sex instinct, being the natural drive for survival of the species, was the prime motivational force of human life. He held that we are born with infinite capacity for sexual expression, and he used the term 'polymorphous-perverse' to describe this potential.

Freud believed that the range of sexual possibilities open to us was far greater than that lived out in everyday practices. His view was that adult patterns of behaviour are based on a blueprint laid down in the earliest years of life. For Freudian theorists, the whole process of civilization consists largely in the 'sublimation' of infantile sexual instinct to other ends than those they seemed designed to serve, so that they are revealed only through the unconscious mind in dreams, fantasies, and jokes. Hence sexuality is always linked with anxiety, stemming from a fear that the banished impulses might break through the barrier of repression. Thus for *Freudian analytic theory*, repression of some sex drives is the cause of psychological disequilibrium and neurosis.

Paradoxically, Freud's own attitude towards many of the forms of sexual behaviour that he claimed so fearlessly to confront, including masturbation, homosexuality, and many aspects of women's sexuality, was one of distaste, leading to contradictions for which his work has been criticized. The constant reference in Freud's work to sexual practices as 'normal' and 'abnormal' is common in the writing of sexologists at the time, and central to the task they set themselves, to comprehensively identify and categorize sexual pathology. Arcane sexual preferences – necrophilia, foot fetishism, nymphomania, for example – were catalogued and described, using terminology such as 'perversions', 'aberrations', and 'deviations'.

Evolutionary psychological and *socio-biological theories* of sexuality also fall into the 'essentialist' camp. Drawing originally on Darwinian theories of evolution, they explain sexuality in terms of reproductive strategies that evolved to ensure survival of the human species (Buss and Schmitt, 1993). According to this perspective, women optimize their chances of passing on their genes by choosing a mate offering the best genetic inheritance for her offspring and living in monogamous union with him, while men optimize theirs by pursuing and impregnating as many women as possible. Most contemporary evolutionary theorists accept that reproduction is no longer the central theme around which modern men and women organize their sexual relations. The sex act is nowadays easily separated from its reproductive consequences by the use of effective contraception, and sexuality has evolved in humans to serve functions other than those solely related to procreation. Yet socio-biology is still used by some to provide an ideological justification for uncontrollable male lust.

Despite their differences, all the early sexologists held a common belief that sex is an overpowering natural force needing either to be contained, channelled, and controlled to allow the orderly working of society, or else released to free us from damaging repressive forces. The preoccupation with sex as driven by biological forces was to last well into the middle of the twentieth century, when Alfred Kinsey's two ground-breaking surveys of the sexual practices of 20,000 men and women in the USA were published (Kinsey et al., 1948, 1953). Kinsey's surveys probably exerted greater influence on ideas about sexuality than any work since that of Sigmund Freud. Yet although he was dismissive of hormones as definitive in explaining sexual response, his approach was still essentially naturalistic. An entomologist by training, Kinsey's scientific interest for the first twenty years of his career was in cataloguing and classifying insects, wasps in particular. When he turned his attention to humans, his attempts to develop a taxonomy of sexual practices very much reflected his background in biology.

Where Kinsey did part company with earlier writers, however, was in moving away from the distinction between 'normal' and 'pathological'. In describing sexual expression in terms of diversity rather than uniformity, Kinsey offered not only an empirical dimension to the study of sexuality, but also a service to the American people. A collective cry of relief is said to have gone up across the USA on publication of the Kinsey report, as thousands of Americans learnt for the first time that personal habits they had previously believed to be shameful, unnatural, and abnormal (such as masturbation), were in fact practised by large numbers of fellow countrymen. Although these ideas still hold sway today, particularly in lay constructions of sexuality, and in certain settings, Kinsey's work did much to remove the categories of 'abnormal' and 'unnatural' from discussions of sexual behaviour.

Sexuality as socially constructed

The alternative way of understanding sexuality – seeing it not as an essentially 'natural' phenomenon, but rather as a product of social and historical forces – began to attract a following in the immediate post-Kinsey era. The sexual diversity hypothesized by Freud from his readings of the unconscious minds of his patients, and demonstrated empirically by Kinsey from his research in the American population, gained further support from the first ever cross-cultural survey of sexual behaviour, undertaken in 1951 (Ford and Beach, 1951). Anthropologists Clellan Ford and Frank Beach showed marked differences in sexual customs from one society to another. In some, the sexual impulses of children were encouraged and allowed expression, in others they were forbidden and punished. Some homosexual activity was considered normal or acceptable in 49 of the 76 societies examined. Different societies held widely different views, rules, and attitudes about sexual exclusiveness; in some societies, non-monogamy was heavily censured, in others polygamy was a normal part of the social arrangements.

Emerging awareness of the marked differences in sexual practices within and between cultures persuaded people that variety, not uniformity, was the norm. Social constructionists pointed to variation between social groups to argue for the cultural relativity of sexual behaviour. If sexuality were solely biologically determined, it was reasoned, then forms of sexual expression would vary little cross-culturally, and the evidence is that they do.

According to this view, there are no universals. A social constructionist approach admits the possibility that the range of sexual possibilities – gender identity, bodily difference, reproductive capacities, needs, desires, and fantasies – may be combined in any number of ways. How we define sex, what counts as sexual, how we code and categorize modes of sexual identity and expression, and what meaning they have in a society, depend on where we live and which era we are born into. Social constructionist theories do not deny the limits imposed by biology or psychology, but their focus is on cultural and social influences as the decisive factors in explaining human sexuality. They contend that our sexual potential and capacities are given meaning only in social relations and through forms of social organization. How we behave sexually is not so much genetically inherited as socially learned, through a variety of discourses. These discourses are embedded in moral treaties, laws, religious strictures, economic policies, educational practices, literature and popular culture, and are acquired through family, peer group, school, the media, and other cultural influences.

Social constructionist theories

One of the first attempts to apply a social constructionist perspective to the study of sexuality was made by John Gagnon and William Simon, whose collaboration began in the late 1960s and led to the publication of their book *Sexual Conduct* (Gagnon and Simon, 1973). Gagnon worked at the Kinsey Institute, but had studied in the Chicago School of Sociology under the influence of George Herbert Mead, who was renowned for formulating the theory of *symbolic interactionism*. Mead held that what distinguishes us from other animals is our wide range of conventional meanings which we express through words and actions. We learn how to adopt and play social roles though the process of 'symbolic interaction', that is, symbolically mediated patterns of reciprocal expectations.

Where Kinsey stopped short of linking sexual variation to social forces and social organization, Gagnon and Simon introduced a systematic interpretation of the social construction of sexual behaviour, one that is embedded in social scripts that are specific to particular cultural and historical settings, vigorously rejecting the determining importance of biological drives or energies. According to *scripting theory*, we use our interactional skills to develop scripts, with cues and appropriate dialogue, as a means of organizing our sexual behaviour. We acquire patterns of sexual conduct that we see as being in keeping with those of our culture or group, but we may make minor individual adaptations to these to fit our own needs and preferences. So while taking account of social-structural factors determining sexual expression, the theory also stresses the significance of individual agency, the idea that an individual is capable of 'making' as well as 'taking' specific social roles and patterns of behaviour.

Other theories are often used in combination with social scripting theory (Laumann et al., 1994). *Choice theory*, for example, focuses on how individuals choose between different options in sexual activities or partnerships according to different goals: sexual pleasure, emotional satisfaction, having children, and enhancing personal reputations. According to this theory, choices made depend on the personal values attached to these goals, the degree of certainty in attaining them, and the factors limiting choice. *Network theory* underlines the dyadic, and therefore essentially social, nature of sexual partnerships and this has three implications (Sprecher and McKinney, 1993). Put simply, people tend to treat their sexual partners in broadly similar ways to others in their social circle; they take account of their partner's action in what they do sexually; and they tend to have sex with the type of individuals they would be likely to have other kinds of relationships with.

Gagnon's work, in turn, paved the way for that of the French critical theorist Michel Foucault. Foucault's *The History of Sexuality* has had a spectacular influence on modern theoretical perspectives, forcing us to rethink our ideas about sexuality and to question the inevitability of the sexual categories and assumptions we have inherited (Foucault, 1983). He focused not only on how sexual conduct changes over time, but on how even the notion of sexuality itself is historically situated. Questions central to Foucault's work include: How and why has sex assumed such importance in Western culture? What is the relationship between sex and power? And how does sexuality relate to economic, social, and political structures?

A balance and a bias

No one theory explains all our sexual behaviour. The kinds of sexual relationships we enter into, the sexual practices we engage in, and the attitudes we hold towards sexuality, all are shaped by a complex network of factors. A comprehensive exploration of sexuality requires an understanding of both biological potential and cultural limits as the preconditions for human sexuality. If innate biological factors were the sole determinants of sexuality, then its expression would vary little between one society and another, yet as we have seen, there are marked differences between sexual norms and customs between different societies. On the other hand, if social factors were all, then members of social subgroups could be expected to exhibit similar forms of sexual behaviour, yet the behaviour of individuals differs even within families. Both sides of the nature–nurture debate help us to understand sexuality and it is also important to recognize both individual agency and social structure when theorizing sexual practices and sexual health outcomes.

Activity 1.1

In pursuing public health goals in relation to sexual health, practitioners often use a social constructionist perspective. Jot down some possible reasons for this.

Feedback

You might have given the following reasons:

Earlier in this chapter we described one of the characterizing features of public health as a focus on the social patterning of behaviours in populations, and on differences between social groups rather than between individuals. Biological and psychological causes may be central when comparing individuals, but this is not the case when comparing groups. Narrowly biological explanations will be inadequate when research questions concern social trends and variations between different populations and subgroups.

You might have noted that theories emphasizing nurture as an influence on behaviour lend themselves better to intervention than do those focussing on nature, since if we are genetically pre-programmed to behave in particular ways there would be little scope for intervening to improve sexual health. Seeing sexual behaviour as fluid rather than fixed offers greater potential for adaptation to changing circumstances and threats, for all the inherent challenges. The aims of public health are less well served by a perspective that is essentially deterministic.

The regulation of sexual behaviour

We have seen that although human sexual capacity is universal, its expression is defined, regulated, and given meaning by cultural norms. Forms of sexual expression vary culturally, but there are neither societies, nor any periods in history, in which there have been no constraints on sexual behaviour. In general, societies support and encourage the kinds of sexual behaviour that best underpin their social arrangements. The raising of stable, well-adjusted children, for example, is seen in most social settings as being best achieved within a monogamous union in a common homestead.

There are some universals. As far as we are aware, there is no society which disapproves of monogamous, heterosexual behaviour aimed at procreation. But societies vary in the extent to which they impose constraints on the polar opposites – notably non-procreative sex, non-exclusive sex, and homosexual behaviour. These are represented diagrammatically in Figure 1.2.

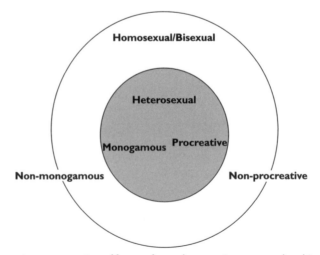

Figure 1.2 A schematic representation of forms of sexual expression commonly subject to social approval and disapproval

Many *non-procreative sexual practices*, for example, have long been the subject of social disapproval or even prohibitive legislation. These include oral and anal sex, same-sex practices, and also sexual activity before the age deemed suitable for childbearing to begin. One of the tenets of the Christian faith – that sex is for reproduction – led to the censorship of practices like oral sex, anal sex, and homosexual sex because they do not lead to pregnancy. The practice of masturbation invokes particularly strong disapproval in this context (Figure 1.3). In the Christian Biblical reference to the sin of Onan in 'spilling' his seed, his transgression was seen as wasting

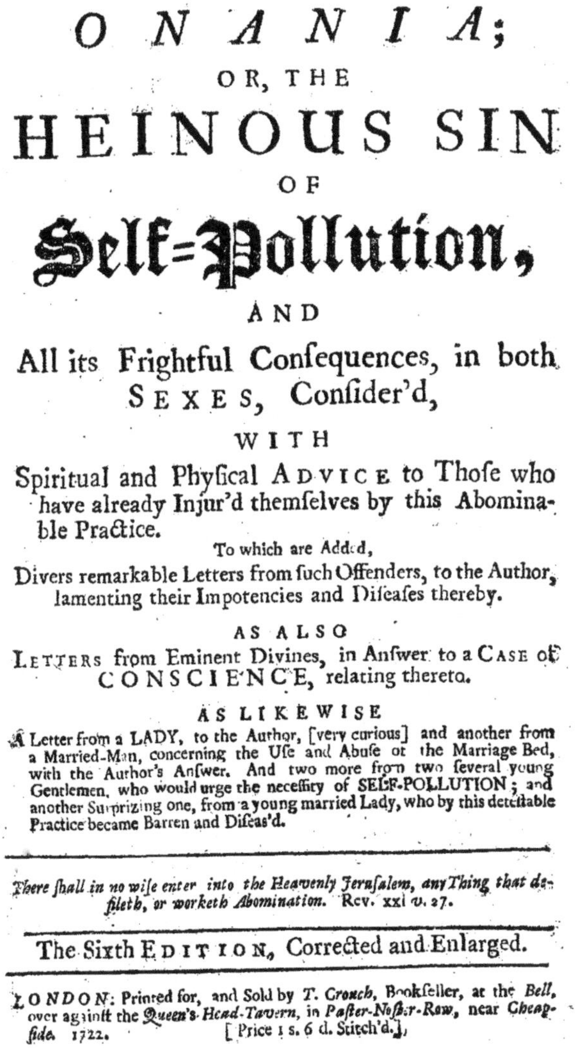

O N A N I A;
OR, THE
HEINOUS SIN
OF
Self=Pollution,
AND
All its Frightful Confequences, in both SEXES, Confider'd,
WITH
Spiritual and Phyfical ADVICE to Thofe who have already Injur'd themfelves by this Abominable Practice.

To which are Added,
Divers remarkable Letters from fuch Offenders, to the Author, lamenting their Impotencies and Difeafes thereby.

AS ALSO
LETTERS from Eminent Divines, in Anfwer to a CASE of CONSCIENCE, relating thereto.

AS LIKEWISE
A Letter from a LADY, to the Author, [very curious] and another from a Married-Man, concerning the Ufe and Abufe of the Marriage Bed, with the Author's Anfwer. And two more from two feveral young Gentlemen, who would urge the neceffity of SELF-POLLUTION ; and another Surprizing one, from a young married Lady, who by this detettable Practice became Barren and Difeas'd.

There fhall in no wife enter into the Heavenly Jerufalem, any Thing that defileth, or worketh Abomination. Rev. xxi v. 27.

The Sixth EDITION, Corrected and Enlarged.

LONDON: Printed for, and Sold by T. Crouch, Bookfeller, at the Bell, over againft the Queen's Head-Tavern, in Pafter-Nofter-Row, near Cheapfide. 1722.   [Price 1 s. 6 d. Stitch'd.]

Figure 1.3 Eighteenth century leaflet warning against masturbation

semen. Vigorous attacks on masturbation were made in the nineteenth century when supposed adverse health implications, including blindness, were used to underpin the moral message.

Activity 1.2

For each of the other two circumscribed areas of sexual expression in Figure 1.2 – that is, non-heterosexual and non-monogamous sex – think of an example of a behaviour that is regulated and describe the way in which constraints have been imposed.

Feedback

In the context of *homosexual sex* (also non-procreative), you might have mentioned the example of sex between men (sex between women has, for the most part, tended to be relatively free from social regulation). Both legal and medical mechanisms have been common forms of control. Until 1861, homosexual behaviour was a hanging offence in England. In America it was not removed from the list of psychiatric disorders until 1973, at which point, as the neuroscientist Simon Levay remarked, '20 million homosexuals gained immediate cure'. (In many countries, homosexuality continues to be regulated legislatively; see Chapter 7.)

You might have chosen as your illustration of how *non-monogamous* sexual relations are regulated, one of the more high-profile instances of public punishments, such as the stoning of 'adulterous' women in some parts of the world. Less extreme examples, however, are far more widespread. In many countries, infidelity almost always constitutes grounds for divorce, and may affect custody of children and the division of property. In addition, many governments create fiscal benefits for men and women who marry.

As the examples in Activity 1.2 show, diverse mechanisms have been used in attempts to regulate sexual behaviour, sometimes in combination. In the past, religion and legislation were commonly invoked. To some extent they still are, though increasing secularization has weakened the hold of religious institutions in many societies and, since sex is largely conducted away from the public gaze, laws are seldom effective in controlling sexual behaviour. Yet the fact that behaviour is illegal may be a powerful assertion of social norms governing the act. A law dating back to 1533 made anal sex between a man and a woman a criminal offence in England and Wales until it was repealed in 2003. In France, where it has never been criminalized, research shows it to be reported twice as commonly as in Britain (Bajos et al., 1995).

In the twenty-first century, medicine and psychology are used to underpin social rules relating to sexuality. Adverse health consequences of sexual behaviour, whether real or not, are often used to deter socially disapproved sexual behaviours. Anti-abortion campaigners in Britain, for example, have claimed links between abortion and breast cancer (Guardian.co.uk; 23 March 2012). And as we shall see in Chapter 2, the threat of sexually transmitted infection is commonly used to deter sexual activity among the young.

Barriers to the improvement of sexual health

Sexual health presents particular challenges for public health. The behaviours involved are not only for the most part personal and private, but are often stigmatized and discriminated against. Morals, taboos, laws, and religious beliefs employed by societies the world over circumscribe and radically determine the sexual behaviour of their citizens. Cross-national comparisons show huge variation in sexual practices. In some countries, such as Brazil, condoms are available to young people in schools; in others, such as parts of Indonesia, possession is a criminal offence. Nowhere are social norms more strongly felt than in the area of homosexual activity. In some parts of the world, sex between men can be celebrated in public parades of pride; in others, it carries the death penalty. Such deterrents may have been put in place to protect wellbeing and rights, yet they can also hinder attempts to protect sexual health. This has consequences for public health at a number of levels.

Activity 1.3

In what ways might the regulation of sexual behaviour impact on public health efforts to improve sexual health?

Feedback

- *Those in need may not come forward for help.* People may not be inclined to seek help for sexual health problems for fear of highlighting that they have been involved in practices that are socially disapproved. Under such circumstances, it would be hard for those involved to access services and interventions.
- *Service providers may not be able to help those in need.* Where behaviours are socially censured, they are often practised covertly and those who do so may be hard to reach in terms of public health efforts. Social attitudes towards harm limitation (such as abortion, provision of contraception to young people, and post-exposure prophylaxis in HIV prevention) also limit service provision.
- *Practitioners may not want to help those in need.* Politicians and even service providers may be unwilling to support provision of services for some populations or may have negative attitudes towards them.
- *Men and women may not be able to help themselves.* Regulation may limit the extent to which men and women can act to protect their health. Stigmatized behaviours may be practised covertly and furtively, making it difficult to talk about and/or practise safer sex.
- *Public health practitioners may not be able to help in ways that they consider to be effective.* Regulation strongly influences the selection of acceptable public health messages and they may be chosen on political rather than scientific grounds.

At this point, you could be thinking that in adopting a social perspective we are doing no more than replacing one form of determinism, deriving from our biological makeup, with another, deriving from the social context. Our genes might not govern our behaviour, but is it not equally strongly dictated by the society in which we live?

To some extent, the answer is possibly 'yes', but in a public health context, we can take a more optimistic view. Social explanations are not inherently deterministic, but instead recognize the duality of agency and structure.

As we have seen, medicine is one of the social forces shaping the expression of sexuality. As such, it can be a conservative or a progressive force. A major challenge for public health lies in confronting existing categories and constraints that act as barriers to the maintenance and improvement of public health. At times, bringing about change in the interests of public health may bring us into conflict with those who would maintain the status quo. Public health has been at the centre of sweeping shifts in recent decades. The lifting of the ban on condom advertising, for example, in France, Britain, and elsewhere in the mid to late 1980s was a direct consequence of the public health response to the advent of the HIV epidemic. Exposure by public health practitioners of the difficulties faced by women in many countries in initiating safer sex practices with partners has brought increasing awareness of gender inequalities and resulted in efforts to address them. At the same time, the public health agenda has been influential in resisting homophobic legislation in Malawi, in Uganda, and most recently in Kenya.

The public health endeavour contributes to the social construction of sexuality and we need to be constantly aware of the ways, often subtle, in which this occurs. We need to be aware, for example, that the language used in a public health context can create or confirm normative categories and serves to maintain distinctions between behaviours that are pathologized and those that are not. We need to be aware that whether we talk of 'drug use' or 'drug misuse', or whether we describe sexual onset in terms such as 'early sex' as opposed to sex before a specified age (see Chapter 6), we are using culturally normative categories and we need to consider the merits and dangers of doing so. We need to be aware that when we talk of categories of people – whether homosexual men or sex workers – we are labelling people rather than describing practices, with all the potential for stigmatization that that affords.

Summary

This book takes a public health approach to sexual behaviour. Guiding the book is a broad definition of sexual health, one that emphasizes not only biomedical goals of averting unplanned pregnancy and sexually transmitted infections, but also behavioural ones such as preventing sexual violence, and which encompasses not only negative but also positive aspects of sexual health, such as wellbeing and satisfaction. Hence, the opening chapters of the book focus on four key areas: unplanned pregnancy, sexually transmitted infections, sexual violence, and sexual function.

We also take a social constructionist approach to sexual health, and so we see sexual behaviour as essentially modifiable. This has two important consequences. First, the fluidity and plasticity of sexuality means that men and women cannot be rigidly pigeonholed in terms of sexual identity, and so for the most part it makes more sense to think in terms of sexual behaviours rather than those practising them. This approach also demands that we take account of social influences on, and regulation of, sexual behaviour and so recognize that to change behaviour requires efforts not only at an individual level, but also at the social structural level. In the search for a healthy lifestyle, a perspective on sexuality that sees opportunities for choice and diversity is more valuable than one that sees sexual behaviour as immutably fixed by biological or psychological forces. A key focus for this book is on the social determinants of sexual health and the social context in which efforts are made to improve it.

References

Bajos N, Wadsworth J, Dudcot B, Johnson AM, Le Pont F, Wellings K et al. (1995) Sexual behaviour in HIV epidemiology: comparative analysis in France and Britain, *AIDS*, 9: 735–43.

Buss DM and Schmitt DP (1993) Sexual strategies theory: an evolutionary perspective on human mating, *Psychological Review*, 100: 204–32.

DeLamater JD and Hyde JS (1998) Essentialism vs. social constructionism in the study of human sexuality, *Journal of Sex Research*, 35: 10–18.

Ford CS and Beach FA (1951) *Patterns of Sexual Behavior*. New York: Harper & Row.

Foucault M (1983) *The History of Sexuality, Vol. 1: The Will to Knowledge*. London: Penguin.

Freud S (1949) *Three Essays on the Theory of Sexuality* (trans. James Strachey). London: Imago Publishing.

Gagnon J and Simon W (1973) *Sexual Conduct: The Social Sources of Human Sexuality*. Chicago, IL: Aldine.

Giami A (2002) Sexual health: the emergence, development, and diversity of a concept, *Annual Review of Sex Research*, 13: 1–35.

Kinsey AA, Pomeroy W and Martin C (1948) *Sexual Behavior in the Human Male*. Philadelphia, PA: WB Saunders.

Kinsey A, Pomeroy W, Martin C and Gebhard P (1953) *Sexual Behavior in the Human Female*. Philadelphia, PA: WB Saunders.

Laumann E, Gagnon JH, Michael RT and Michaels S (1994) *The Social Organization of Sexuality: Sexual Practices in the United States*. Chicago, IL: University of Chicago Press.

MacDougall H (2007) Reinventing public health: a new perspective on the health of Canadians and its international impact, *Journal of Epidemiology and Community Health*, 61: 955–9.

Sandfort TGM and Ehrhardt AA (2004) Sexual health: a useful public health paradigm or a moral imperative?, *Archives of Sexual Behaviour*, 33(3): 181–7.

Sprecher S and McKinney K (1993) *Sexualities*. London: Sage.

Weeks J (2003) *Sexuality*, rev. 2nd edn. London: Routledge.

World Health Organization (WHO) (2006) *Defining Sexual Health: Report of a Technical Consultation on Sexual Health*, 28–31 January 2002. Geneva: WHO. Available at: http://www.who.int/reproductive-health/publications/sexualhealth/index.html (accessed 31 January 2012).

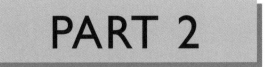

PART 2

Sexual health outcomes

Sexually transmitted infections

2

Kaye Wellings, Sevgi O. Aral,
Jami Leichliter and Thomas Peterman

Overview

Sexually transmitted infections (STIs) are possibly the most familiar adverse outcomes of sexual activity and are among the most common causes of ill health in the world. In this chapter, you will learn about the distribution of the most common STIs and their moral and medical significance. You will also gain an understanding of the factors affecting prevalence and transmission, and the implications of this knowledge for STI prevention and control.

Learning outcomes

After reading this chapter, you will be able to:

- Understand the impact of STI on global ill health
- Identify the range of determinants of STI transmission
- Appreciate the challenges in explaining change over time, and variation across settings, in STI prevalence and transmission
- Explain the need for a broadly based and multi-faceted approach to STI control

Key terms

Incidence rate: The rate at which new infections occur in a population. The numerator is the number of new events occurring in a defined period; the denominator is the population at risk of experiencing the event during the chosen period (most commonly a year).

Infectivity: The attributes of an individual or pathogen likely to lead to spread of infection.

Prevalence: The proportion of individuals in a population with an infection or disease at any one time.

Prophylaxis: Measures designed to preserve health and prevent the spread of disease: protective or preventive treatment against infection.

Susceptibility: The attribute(s) of an individual likely to make them more or less likely to be affected by infection or disease.

Introduction

The category sexually transmitted infections (STIs) refers to a diverse range of pathogens that manifest themselves in a number of ways. Some are minor irritations, whereas others can be fatal. Sexually transmitted infections include: bacterial infections, such as gonorrhoea (*Neisseria gonorrhoeae*), chlamydia (*Chlamydia trachomatis*), chancroid, and syphilis; viral infections, such as human immunodeficiency virus (HIV), human papilloma virus, herpes simplex virus, human cytomegalovirus, hepatitis B, and *Mycoplasma genitalium*; parasites, such as crabs; and protozoal infections, such as trichomoniasis. The common factor in all these infections is their primary mode of transmission and acquisition. An STI is an infection that has a higher probability of transmission via sexual contact than by any other means.

Until the 1990s, STIs were commonly known as venereal diseases, after Venus, the Roman goddess of love. Social disease was another euphemism. The term 'sexually transmitted infection' is now commonly used in public health, in preference to the term 'sexually transmitted disease', since many STIs (e.g. HIV, chlamydia, human papilloma virus) exhibit no signs or symptoms of disease for some time after acquisition, if ever. This is important in a public health context, since STIs are often transmitted by people who are unaware they are infected.

The list of STIs is constantly growing, as 'new' infections are added. Sexually transmitted infections such as chlamydia, human papilloma virus, and *Mycoplasma genitalium* have only recently been identified. Others have a far longer history. Although the start of the HIV/AIDS epidemic is usually dated from 1979, when the first death from the infection occurred in the USA, laboratory analysis of blood samples has revealed the existence of HIV infection more than half a century ago. Herpes has been known for at least 2000 years. In ancient Rome, the emperor Tiberius banned kissing, so serious was the epidemic of lip sores, and Shakespeare refers to 'blisters oe'r ladies lips' in 'Romeo and Juliet'. The first European outbreak of syphilis was recorded in 1494, among French troops besieging Naples, yet scientists have found evidence of skeletal destruction associated with syphilis in bone remains carbon-dated to before the fifteenth century in parts of the new world.

Sex, sickness, and sin

An individual gets an STI not because he or she has sex, but through sexual contact with an infected person. Nevertheless, in attempts to regulate and control sexual behaviour, the threat of STIs has long been used as a deterrent to any sexual activity. Sexually transmitted infections are often described in terms of retribution and punishment for sin and references to the 'wages of sin' and 'the price of love' are common (Allen, 2000). And distinctions tend to be made between 'guilty' and 'innocent' victims according to whether the infection was acquired by sexual or non-sexual means (for example, through infected blood or mother-to-child transmission). The notion of retribution in relation to STI acquisition has consequences both for the development and provision of therapeutic remedies, since the belief that disease is a just desert for moral transgression is common.

Because of the negative moral connotations of STIs, the tendency through history has been to see them as afflictions of 'the other'. When an epidemic of syphilis was first described in fifteenth-century Italy following the French invasion, it was described as the 'French disease', and when the city of Shanghai was still under European control during the early twentieth century, the Chinese held syphilis to be an import brought by the Portuguese. The tendency to distance oneself from people at risk of STIs continues today, and manifests in a reluctance to associate with what are seen as stereotypical characteristics of infected persons, in terms of illicit sex and moral transgression. Since pathogens themselves make no moral distinctions, the tendency to distance oneself from risk of STI has negative consequences for public health.

The burden of disease

Sexually transmitted infections represent a major burden of disease. Prevalence and incidence remain high in most of the world, despite therapeutic advances. Estimates are limited by the quantity and quality of data available, but the WHO puts the number of new cases of selected, curable STIs worldwide in 2005 at nearly 500 million (Camaroni et al., 2012).

The global prevalence of adults living with HIV has been unchanged since 2000 at 0.8%. However, the estimated number of people living with HIV increased from 29.5 million in 2001 to 33.4 million in 2008. In 2008, 70% of new HIV infections and HIV-related deaths occurred in sub-Saharan Africa and HIV is the single largest cause of mortality in the region. HIV/AIDS is also the leading cause of death among African-American women aged 25–34 years (van Dam, 2012).

Sexually transmitted infections have far-reaching health, social, and economic consequences. Complications can be serious and are found more often in resource-poor settings, and within countries among the poor. Sexually transmitted infections also disproportionately affect the heath and wellbeing of women, particularly those in the reproductive age range. In women, STIs can lead to pelvic inflammatory disease, chronic pelvic pain, ectopic pregnancy, and infertility. In both men and women, untreated STIs can result in infertility, cancers and, in the case of syphilis, neurological and heart disease.

Understanding the determinants of STI transmission

An understanding of the factors influencing the prevalence of STIs in a population, and their likely pace of spread, is essential to STI control. Mathematical models of STI transmission dynamics describe the reproductive rate of an STI, or its potential for spread in a population, according to the equation:

$$R_0 = \beta \times c \times D,$$

where R_0 is the reproductive rate and is determined by β, the likelihood of transmission between an infected and a susceptible individual; c, the rate of contact between infected and susceptible individuals; and D, the length of time a person remains infected (Garnett, 2008). When R_0 is greater than one, the infection will continue to spread and incidence will increase; when R_0 is smaller than one, the incidence is reducing and the infection will disappear from the population. The aim of all prevention and control strategies is to reduce R_0 to less than one, and therefore to address the determinants β, c, and D.

Activity 2.1

What do you think some of these determinants might be?

Feedback

A complex web of biological, behavioural, and social factors influences the likelihood of STI transmission. Those you noted may have fallen into the following categories:

- *Biomedical and epidemiological factors*: for example, characteristics of the infection; prevalence rates in a particular setting; the susceptibility of the non-infected person and the infectivity of the infected person.
- *Behavioural factors*: for example, sexual practices, partnerships, and risk-reduction strategies.
- *Health service-related factors*: for example, willingness to seek health care and to report STI symptoms; access to services and the quality of health care.
- *Social contextual factors*: for example, level of resources in a setting; attitudes towards prevention and treatment; social norms and laws relating to STIs.

These are dealt with in more detail in the following subsections.

Biomedical factors

The probability of transmission of an STI is influenced by the organism involved, the part of the body it enters, and the integrity of the skin or mucosal barrier. Rates of transmission are generally estimated from studies of discordant couples, in which one person is infected and the other is not (though couples where transmission has not already occurred may be atypical in important ways). Such trials have been conducted for HIV and herpes where infections are chronic. Bacterial infections are less easily studied, but data have been obtained from studies of partner notification.

Infection rates vary by infectious organism. For example, while the estimated risk of transmission of HIV per single sexual contact is 0.04% for women-to-men and 0.08% for men-to-women (Holmes et al., 2008; Boily et al., 2009), for gonorrhoea it is 20% for men following a single contact with an infected woman (Holmes et al., 2008). How easily infections can pass from one person to another also depends on their stage. Herpes, for example, is much more likely to spread when blisters are present.

Infectivity and susceptibility are also influenced by behavioural factors. The integrity of skin and mucous membranes of the body can be weakened by the practice of douching, the use of astringents, or by co-infections causing breaks and abrasions in the skin, which provide a portal of entry for other infectious organisms. Alternatively, integrity can be reinforced and defended, by circumcision for instance, and by the use of condoms or chemical barriers such as spermicides.

Ulceration and lesions of the skin caused by the presence of one STI allow an entry point for others. This is more common in developing countries, either because STIs are less well treated or because, as in the case of chancroid, they are largely restricted to those settings. A host of epidemiological studies has suggested that STIs are co-factors for HIV acquisition or transmission, the most reliable of which suggest a 2.6-fold increase in risk of HIV transmission if the HIV-infected partner also has genital ulceration (Gray et al., 2001). Thus treatment for one STI can, in itself, be a protective strategy in relation to possible infection with another STI (see Chapter 14 for a description of the syndromic management of STIs).

Behavioural factors

Sexual practices

How easily infections can be acquired varies by sexual practice. HIV is more easily transmitted through anal than vaginal sex, possibly because anal mucosa is more susceptible than vaginal mucosa, and is rarely acquired through oral sex. Syphilis, by contrast, can be transmitted via oral sex, and so a switch from anal to oral sex among men who have sex with men reduces transmission for HIV, but may have little if any effect on the transmission of syphilis (Holmes et al., 2008).

Risk-reduction strategies

Male condoms are the first line of defence in preventing STIs and, in theory, can substantially reduce risk of infection. Meta-analyses of cohorts of discordant couples have shown consistent condom use to reduce HIV transmission by 80–95% (Holmes et al., 2008). In practice, correct and consistent condom use is uncommon. Many people use condoms for a short while after meeting a new partner, and then stop, or else use them intermittently. Condoms are less commonly used in poorer countries, which is likely attributable to factors relating to access and service provision (Wellings et al., 2006). Not surprisingly, condoms are more effective in preventing infections transmitted through genital fluids, such as gonorrhoea, chlamydia, hepatitis B, and HIV, than those transmitted from ulcers or warts situated in areas that a condom would not cover.

The capacity of female barrier methods to halt the spread of STIs has been disappointing. Some studies have found an increased risk of acquiring HIV, possibly due to irritation of the delicate genital membranes providing a portal of entry for the virus. Yet a recent trial found that a vaginal gel reduced the risk of HIV and herpes simplex virus by up to 50%, giving hope that more effective microbicide gels could be identified (Abdool Karim et al., 2010).

Male circumcision

One of the most striking pieces of evidence to emerge in recent years in relation to STI prevention is the protective effect of male circumcision. However, the protection is only partial (Weiss et al., 2010); randomized trials have shown circumcision to reduce transmission to men via penile–vaginal sex by 50–60% for HIV, 30–45% for herpes simplex virus 2, and 30% for human papilloma virus. Moreover, the trials found no clear decrease in transmission from men to women and as yet there is no information on the effect of circumcision on transmission between men who have sex with men. Access to safe circumcision services together with behavioural counselling is still needed (Larke and Weiss, 2012).

Partnerships and partner change

Multiple sexual partnerships increase the risk of STIs and HIV. Risk of infection increases for both men and women with number of sexual partners (Gouveia-Oliveira and Pedersen, 2009), and a woman's risk is also significantly increased if her partner has multiple partners (Canchihuaman et al., 2010).

Epidemiologists distinguish between multiple partnerships that occur *serially* (i.e. one begins after another has ended) and those that occur *concurrently* (i.e. a man or woman has other sexual partners while continuing sexual activity with the original partner). Until recently, concurrent partnerships were widely believed to play a role in accelerating the spread of STIs (Gorbach and Holmes, 2003; Senn et al., 2009), but this view is now contested (Aral, 2010; Kretzschmar et al., 2010). Short gaps between serially monogamous partners may have the same effect where partner change occurs while STIs are still infectious. Emerging evidence from sub-Saharan Africa rebuts the idea that concurrent partnerships are an important driver of HIV incidence, concluding that risk is not affected by whether those partnerships overlap in time (Tanser et al., 2011).

Sexual networks and sexual mixing patterns

Sexual mixing patterns are described as *assortative*, where sexual contact is between individuals with similar social and behavioural characteristics, and *dissortative*, where sexual contact is between individuals with dissimilar characteristics. Assortative mixing has a lower potential for spread of STIs where sexual contact is between individuals at similarly low risk, but can result in initially rapid spread where sexual contact is between those with large numbers of sexual partners. Dissortative mixing, where sex occurs between partners of unequal risk status, is likely to lead to greater spread, though more slowly.

Age mixing – that is, sexual contact between a younger and an older partner – may be an important determinant of STI/HIV prevalence in young people. This pattern is common in some countries in Africa, where young people greatly outnumber older people, and where many older men have sex with younger women. Median age differences between partners in Africa are comparatively large.

Individuals with the highest rates of partner change contribute disproportionately to the spread of STIs and are often described as constituting the *core group*. Sexual contact between members of the core group and individuals with fewer sexual contacts facilitates STI transmission in populations, and may be high enough to sustain STI transmission within the larger population.

Health service provision and use

Prompt and effective treatment of sexually transmitted diseases plays a key role in curbing the spread of infection in populations, by reducing the duration of infection and so reducing the number of infectious individuals (van Dam, 2012). The extent to which optimal treatment is possible in practice reflects a number of factors.

Foremost among these is the availability of a therapeutic remedy. This varies according to pathogen, but enormous progress has been made in the area of STI and HIV prophylaxis in recent decades. The discovery of penicillin in 1943 represented a momentous advance in STI control. Treatment of bacterial infections had been possible since Paul Ehrlich's discovery of salvarsan (an organic arsenic compound) in 1909, but was lengthy, painful, and had side effects. An equally significant advance was the introduction of highly active anti-retroviral therapy (HAART) in 1995, a combination of powerful protease inhibitors with other HIV medications. Anti-retroviral therapy has been shown to hugely diminish the chances of transmission of HIV by an infected person, by 96%. This has subsequently been augmented by pre-exposure and post-exposure prophylaxis in the treatment of HIV. A protective vaccine against hepatitis B (HBV) has been available for many years, and in 2006 a vaccine against the most common carcinogenic strain of human papilloma virus was approved for use in the UK, the USA, and elsewhere. Treatment is available for herpes in the form of acyclovir.

There are exceptions to this forward march. A vaccine offering protection against HIV has been elusive and the development and spread of drug-resistant bacteria (penicillin-resistant gonococci) makes some STIs more difficult to cure. But in general therapeutic advances have been so spectacular that some are talking in terms of minimization of duration of infectiousness and viral load becoming the most potent intervention for prevention of HIV spread in populations.

A cautionary note is needed in this context. The availability of sophisticated medications is regionally highly variable. Problems of access severely limit their therapeutic potential, particularly in poorer countries and in those in which the political will to prioritize provision is lacking. Challenges also relate to adherence, most notably in the case of HAART.

Delays in treatment result from failure to seek health care on the part of those in need. Many STIs are often asymptomatic and where there are symptoms they are not always recognized by those affected. This is compounded by fears and hesitation on the part of patients. Delays may also result from the provision of sub-optimal health care. Waiting times at clinics may be long, and diagnosis often flawed. Problems of communication are common; both physicians and patients have difficulty dealing openly and candidly with sexual issues (see Chapter 11). A study in South Africa showed that 25% of women surveyed were infected with an STI, of whom 48% were asymptomatic, 50% were symptomatic but not seeking care, 1.7% were symptomatic and would seek care, while only 0.3% were actually seeking care the day they were surveyed (van Dam, 2012). Such findings underscore the importance of a holistic, comprehensive approach to STI and HIV prevention and control.

The question of whether the availability of a cure for STI makes people more likely to engage in sexually risky behaviours by removing the deterrent of fear of infection crops up repeatedly in discussions of STI control. It resonates with the argument adopted by some opponents of contraception, namely that it removes the fear of unwanted pregnancy and so endorses sexual risk-taking behaviour. While there is some evidence that the introduction of HAART was followed by a period characterized by what became known as 'relapse' among gay men, marked by a return to higher levels of risky behaviours, few would deny that the net benefits of HAART have far outweighed any unintended outcomes.

Social and political conditions affecting STI transmission

Marked changes in sexual behaviour in the past half century have influenced the transmission of STIs. To an extent, these have occurred in response to demographic changes, in the age structures of populations (e.g. in the timing of marriage), and in the size of families. Attitudes towards sexual behaviour have also changed significantly in recent times. Global forms of communication, including the Internet, have had a bearing on social norms, transporting Western sexual images to more conservative societies, particularly those in which advances in information technology have been rapid.

Historically, STIs flourish in conditions of maximum mixing of populations and the scale of mobility and migration between and within countries has increased. The effect of travel is most dramatically illustrated by the rapid spread of HIV from Africa to Europe and the Americas in the late 1970s (see Chapter 9). The increases in intra- and international travel have played their part in increasing possibilities for the transmission of STIs, but so too have changing patterns of labour involving rural to urban movement.

Social disruption due to war and political instabilities also increases STI transmission rates. Wars lead to liaisons between mercenaries and soldiers and members of local populations, and often impact on rape and prostitution. Wars are also characterized by social upheaval, population mobility and displacement, and unequal power relations between occupied and occupier. The immediate aftermath of war is characterized by the break up of stable relationships.

Gender roles and inequities, and power relations in sexual relationships, also contribute to increased probability of STI transmission (see Chapter 10). Many women, for instance, are aware that they are at risk of acquiring an STI or HIV infection from partners but are not in a situation to safely and effectively negotiate condom use. Women's power to maintain monogamous relationships might be diminished in settings in which they outnumber men with whom they might have sex. Imbalances in the number of women to men may result from the age structures of populations and patterns of age mixing, from cultural practices such as polygyny, and from high levels of imprisonment of black men distorting sex ratios in predominantly African-American communities, as in the USA (Adimora and Schoenbach, 2002).

Understanding changes in STI prevalence over time

From the overview of the determinants of STI prevalence and transmission above, we can see that the influences on STI transmission are multiple, and that there is considerable interaction between them.

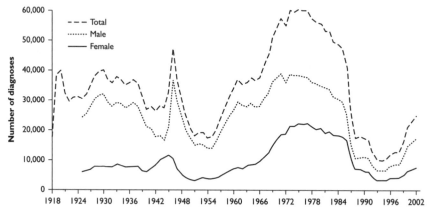

Figure 2.1 Diagnoses of gonorrhoea seen in genitourinary medicine clinics, England and Wales, 1918–2002. Data for Scotland and Northern Ireland excluded, because they are incomplete for the period shown
Source: KC60/HPA

Activity 2.2

Study Figure 2.1, which shows the numbers of diagnosed cases of gonorrhoea in England and Wales over the past century and more. What trends do you observe and what might be the possible reasons for these?

Feedback

You may have made some preliminary observations. First, the graph charts numbers and not rates, and we need to take account of the fact that the population of England and Wales doubled during the century represented. We could therefore expect gonorrhoea rates, if all else had remained constant, to do the same. Second, the choice of gonorrhoea to demonstrate trends is unavoidable from the point of view of providing robust data and a lengthy historical span, but it is not necessarily a good proxy for trends in other STIs. Finally, diagnoses will reflect health care attendances, and the trend is likely to have been towards greater willingness to report symptoms and seek treatment over a period in which the stigma of an STI lessened.

That said, you may have noted the increases in gonorrhoea diagnoses, higher for men but discernible for women, coinciding with the First World War (1914–18) and Second World War (1939–45). The figures fell again immediately after both wars, though more dramatically after the Second World War, to lower than pre-war values. The subsequent rise in gonorrhoea diagnoses, from the mid-1950s to the mid-1970s, is more gradual, but of greater magnitude. We then see a strikingly steep decline in diagnoses during the 1980s, to values that are the lowest of the century, followed by a slight upturn dating from the mid-1990s.

How do we explain the fluctuations? As we saw in our discussion of the determinants of STI transmission, we might expect increases in STI incidence during wartime. But the peak associated with the Second World War coincides not only with wartime but with the discovery, in 1943, of penicillin as an effective therapy for syphilis and gonorrhoea. In fact, the outbreak of the Second World War provided the impetus for research into a cure, since STIs accounted for a substantial number of days of active service lost. Did access to effective treatment increase the number of gonorrhoea diagnoses? Or was it the wartime effect? The combined influence of these factors on sexual behaviour and STI transmission makes it difficult to disentangle the effects of a 'cure' from features of the wartime period, though one telling fact is that rates of gonorrhoea also increased during the First World War, when there was no 'antibiotic effect'.

It is equally difficult to provide a single explanation for the rise in gonorrhoea diagnoses from the mid-1950s to the mid-1970s. The decades following the Second World War in England were a time of liberalizing reform in the legislation governing sexual behaviour, and this coincided with a period of softening attitudes and greater sexual freedom. The existence of a cure for bacterial STIs led to a public perception during the 1960s that they had ceased to be a serious medical threat, and with the advent of effective anti-microbial agents in the 1950s and 1960s, STI control efforts focused for the most part on clinical care with little attention paid to behavioural interventions.

Given the timing, it is difficult to attribute the very steep decline in gonorrhoea rates during the 1980s to other than the effect of the advent of the HIV/AIDS epidemic, particularly on risk reduction practice, notably condom use. The amount of publicity, both in the free media and in paid-for government campaigns, was unprecedented. Not until the twenty-first century did the figures begin to climb again, and even then to nowhere near the levels seen earlier in the century.

Understanding differences in STI prevalence across settings

The factors explaining differences across settings are equally difficult to fathom. We still do not fully understand the regional variability in the speed and extent of STI and HIV transmission. Epidemiological studies in Africa, for example, have observed little association between respondents' self-reported sexual behaviour and their HIV status (Buvé et al., 2012). Several studies have shown an absence of correlation between risk behaviour and STIs prevalence. Such puzzling findings have led some to search for less obvious explanations for the African AIDS epidemic.

Activity 2.3

Figure 2.2 shows the global distribution for age-standardized, disability-adjusted life years (DALYs) for STIs (excluding HIV) per 100,000 inhabitants in 2004. A DALY is calculated to represent one lost year of 'healthy' life, and is a useful measure of the burden of disease attributable to a particular health condition. What do you note about their distribution globally? What factors might explain the distribution?

Feedback

Figure 2.2 shows fairly unequivocally that STIs impact most in the poorest countries of the world. The highest DALY scores are found in the poorer countries of Africa and in South Asia, the lowest in the richer countries of North America, Europe, North Asia, and Australia. In terms of a behavioural explanation, this appears counterintuitive. Global comparisons of sexual behaviour (Wellings et al., 2006) show that the prevalence of multiple partnerships and premarital sex varies regionally but is notably higher in the richer countries in which STIs are less prevalent.

In searching for an explanation, you may have questioned whether the data on sexual behaviour were reliable, and whether underestimates of risk practices might account for the apparent paradox of higher rates of STIs and lower rates of multiple partnerships. Most methodological reviews of research into sexual behaviour have revealed that the validity and reliability of data may be lower in developing countries.

Alternatively, it may have occurred to you that the answer might lie in the prevalence of risk reduction practice, as opposed to risk behaviour. The prevalence of condom use is significantly lower in resource-poor countries (Wellings et al., 2006) and this may be associated with access, difficulties faced by women in asserting the need for condom use, and social norms militating against use, including those prioritizing fertility over prevention of infection.

In identifying explanations other than those relating to sexual behaviour, an obvious one, perhaps, is health care. The likelihood of prompt medical attention and effective treatment is lower in poorer, and more rural, countries, and so the duration of infection is likely to be longer. In this context, the impact of co-factors is likely to be relevant. Untreated genital ulcers and sores weakening the defences against further STI transmission are likely to be more common.

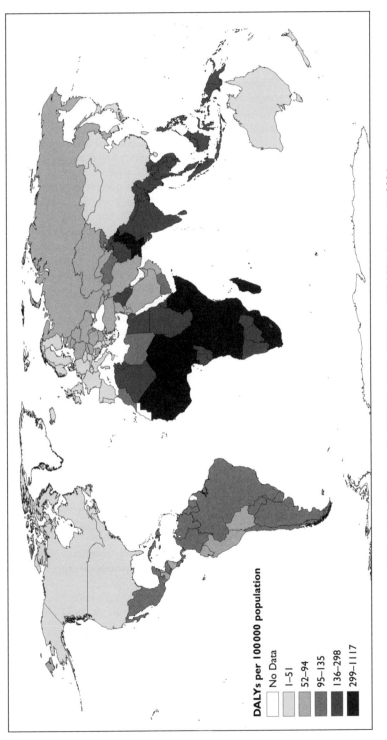

DALYs per 100000 population

No Data
1–51
52–94
95–135
136–298
299–1117

Figure 2.2 Age-standardized, disability-adjusted life years for STIs (excluding HIV) per 100,000 inhabitants in 2004

Source: WHO disease and injury country estimates, 2004

The scope for intervention

Efforts to control STIs have evolved over time and continue to do so. Before the advent of effective therapies, containment and control, supported by quarantine and legal constraints, was the most common approach. During the nineteenth century, efforts to control STIs by regulating prostitution gave widespread authority to police officers to arrest women merely on suspicion of prostitution. In the Second World War, the acquisition of an STI was a crime subject to loss of pay in some countries. Legislative mechanisms were still being used in STI control at the start of the HIV epidemic. In the 1980s, countries such as Sweden and Cuba segregated those people with HIV who were thought to pose a threat of infection to others. Still today, the act of intentionally infecting others is a criminal offence in many countries.

The use of legislation in STI control has, however, become increasingly less common. In the 1990s, containment and control measures gave way to communication and persuasion as means of raising awareness of HIV/AIDS, demolishing myths and providing pointers to preventive action. The emergence of new incurable viral STIs, especially HIV, underscored prevention efforts focused on the individual, promoting safer sexual behaviour and the use of barrier methods. These are still in sway in high prevalence areas but with increasing recognition of the importance of the social, cultural, and economic determinants of behaviour (see Chapter 12). Few countries have successfully overcome the social, cultural, religious and, above all, resource constraints to reducing STI prevalence. In the absence of an enabling and supportive environment, many individuals may be unable or unwilling to adopt safer behaviours.

The contemporary spirit seems, by some accounts, to be swinging back in favour of an emphasis on vaccines and cures. Yet enthusiasm for the therapeutic option needs to be tempered by recall of the upsurge in STIs in the 1970s, when treatment was not accompanied by advice on risk reduction. Treatment options still do not exist for all STIs. Where they do, they are not always accessed promptly, are not adhered to by all, and are not effective in every case. The maxim that 'all drugs are useful poisons' is apt in this context. Such is the toxicity and unpleasantness of many medications that few would argue seriously in favour of treatment replacing prevention.

A mix of STI control strategies is needed. Therapies are not foolproof, and they depend on identifying people at risk and motivating them to come forward for treatment. Therapies also tend to be specific to particular groups of STIs and the possibility of new infections emerging for which there is no cure has recent precedent. The history of STI control teaches us the importance of sustaining efforts to raise awareness and support behavioural strategies to reduce risk. When, in the 1980s, HIV/AIDS emerged into the public consciousness as a sexually transmitted infection that could not be cured by modern medicine, it caught out a generation unpractised in the art of risk reduction.

For maximum impact, STI and HIV control programmes require a variety of approaches tailored to the prevalence in the population, the social and cultural context, the availability of resources, and the priority accorded this area of health care by policy-makers. A combination of both individual and population level approaches is crucial in the case of communicable diseases, since individual interventions are likely to have an effect at the population level.

At the level of health service provision, high-quality clinical services are needed to reduce the prevalence of curable STIs. Integrating STIs with other sexual health services may reduce the stigma that prevents people from seeking help (see Chapter 14) and efforts are needed to address pejorative attitudes of health care staff. As discussed, recent findings have underscored the importance of pre-exposure prophylaxis as well as early treatment in the primary prevention of HIV. Contact tracing, locating the sexual partners of infected individuals, testing and treating them for infection, and in turn tracing their contacts, continues to be an important measure, even when diseases are incurable, as it helps to contain infection.

Educational interventions aimed at reducing the risk of infection through the adoption and maintenance of safer sex behaviours will continue to be needed. There is a need for straightforward, unambiguous messages aimed at the reduction of multiple partnerships, irrespective of whether they overlap in time, and at consistent condom use. Multi-level approaches are required for successful prevention programmes, addressing both individual behaviours as well as the social context.

Summary

Sexually transmitted infections comprise a major health burden globally. To understand the prevalence and distribution of STIs in a population and their likely pace of spread, we need to consider the characteristics of the infectious agents, the range of sexual behaviours in a population, the availability and quality of treatment services, the wider social and cultural environment, and the nature and effectiveness of preventive efforts. The links between patterns of sexual behaviour in a population and rates of spread of STIs are variable and complex. Successful prevention of STIs requires a combination of individual and population level approaches that focus on reducing the risk of transmission.

Disclaimer

The findings and conclusions in this paper are those of the authors and do not necessarily represent the views of the Centers for Disease Control and Prevention.

References

Abdool Karim QA, Abdool Karim SS, Frohlich JA, Grobler AC, Baxter C, Mansoor LE et al. (2010) Trial effectiveness and safety of Tenofovir gel, an antiretroviral microbicide, for the prevention of HIV infection in women, *Science*, 329(5996): 1168–74.

Adimora AA and Schoenbach VJ (2002) Contextual factors and the black–white disparity in heterosexual HIV transmission, *Epidemiology*, 13: 707–12.

Allen PL (2000) *The Wages of Sin: Sex and Disease Past and Present*. Chicago, IL: University of Chicago Press.

Aral SO (2010) Partner concurrency and the STD/HIV epidemic, *Current Infectious Disease Reports*, 12: 134–9.

Boily MC, Baggaley RF, Wang L, Masse B, White RG, Hayes RJ et al. (2009) Heterosexual risk of HIV-1 infection per sexual act: systematic review and meta-analysis of observational studies. *Lancet Infectious Diseases*, 9: 118–29.

Buvé A, Bishikwabo-NsarhazaAli H, Micalef J and Donovan B (2012) Global epidemiology of HIV infection, in S. Gupta and B. Kumar (eds.) *Sexually Transmitted Infections*, 2nd edn. New Delhi: Elsevier.

Camaroni I, Toskin I, Ndowa F and Gerbase AC (2012) Global epidemiology of sexually transmitted infections, in S. Gupta and B. Kumar (eds.) *Sexually Transmitted Infections*, 2nd edn. New Delhi: Elsevier.

Canchihuaman FA, Carcamo CP, Garcia PJ, Aral SO, Whittington WLH, Hawes SE et al. (2010) Non-monogamy and risk of infection with *Chlamydia trachomatis* and *Trichomonas vaginalis* among young adults and their partners in Peru, *Sexually Transmitted Infections*, 86(suppl. 3): iii37–iii44.

Garnett GP (2008) The transmission dynamics of sexually transmitted infections, in KK Holmes, PF Sparling, WE Stamm, P Piot, JN Wasserheit, L Corey (eds.) *Sexually Transmitted Diseases*, 4th edn. New York: McGraw-Hill Medical.

Gorbach PM and Holmes KK (2003) Transmission of STIs/HIV at the partnership level: beyond individual-level analyses. *Journal of Urban Health*, 80: iii15–iii25.

Gouveia-Oliveira R and Pedersen AG (2009) Higher variability in the number of sexual partners in males can contribute to a higher prevalence of sexually transmitted diseases in females, *Journal of Theoretical Biology*, 261: 100–6.

Gray RH, Wawer MJ, Brookmeyer R, Sewankambo NK, Serwadda D, Wabwire-Mangen F et al. (2001) Probability of HIV-1 transmission per coital act in monogamous, heterosexual, HIV-1-discordant couples in Rakai, Uganda, *Lancet*, 357: 1149–53.

Holmes KK, Sparling PF, Stamm WE, Piot P, Wasserheit JN, Corey L et al. (eds.) (2008) *Sexually Transmitted Diseases*, 4th edn. New York: McGraw-Hill Medical.

Kretzschmar M, White RG and Caraël M (2010) Concurrency is more complex than it seems, *AIDS*, 24: 313–15.

Senn TE, Carey MP, Vanable PA, Coury-Doniger P and Urban M (2009) Sexual partner concurrency among STI clinic patients with a steady partner: correlates and associations with condom use, *Sexually Transmitted Infections*, 85: 343–7.

Tanser F, Bärnighausen T, Hund L, Garnett GP, McGrath N and Newell M-L (2011) Effect of concurrent sexual partnerships on rate of new HIV infections in a high-prevalence, rural South African population: a cohort study, *Lancet*, 378(9787): 247–55.

van Dam J (2012) Prevention strategies for the control of sexually transmitted infections, in S. Gupta and B. Kumar (eds.) *Sexually Transmitted Infections*, 2nd edn. New Delhi: Eslevier.

Weiss HA, Dickson KE, Agot K and Hankins CA (2010) Male circumcision for HIV prevention: current research and programmatic issues, *AIDS*, 24(suppl. 4): S61–S69.

Weiss H and Larke NL (2012) Prevention of Sexually Transmitted Infections and HIV: Male circumcision in S. Gupta and B. Kumar (eds) *Sexually Transmitted Infections*, 2nd edn. New Delhi: Elsevier.

Wellings K, Collumbien M, Slaymaker E, Singh S, Hodges Z, Patel D et al. (2006) Sexual behaviour in context: a global perspective, *Lancet*, 368(9548): 1706–28.

Further reading

Davidson R and Hall LA (eds.) (2001) *Sex, Sin and Suffering: Venereal Disease and European Society since 1870*. New York: Routledge (pp. 220–36).

Unplanned pregnancy

Anna Glasier and Kaye Wellings

Overview

Unplanned pregnancy has the potential to impact negatively on women's lives by restricting their opportunities and perpetuating cycles of poverty. In this chapter, we explore the meaning and measurement of unplanned pregnancy and its prevalence and consequences. We examine the challenges in improving the uptake, continuation, and correct use of contraception and the benefits of doing so for men and women, and for society.

Learning outcomes

After reading this chapter, you will be able to:

- Discuss the meaning of unplanned pregnancy and understand issues relating to its measurement
- Describe global patterns of unplanned pregnancy, and their causes and consequences
- Recognize the factors that influence the uptake, choice, continuation, and effective use of contraception
- Identify potential directions for effective public health intervention to reduce unplanned pregnancy

Key terms

Abortion: The termination of pregnancy by the removal or expulsion from the womb of a foetus or embryo prior to viability. A spontaneous abortion is termed a 'miscarriage'. The term 'abortion' most commonly refers to induced termination of a pregnancy where this is intentional.

Emergency contraception: This is a term used to describe the use of a drug or device after intercourse to prevent pregnancy.

Unmet need: Women who are sexually active but not using contraception, and who do not want a child within two years, are considered to have an 'unmet need' for family planning.

Unsafe abortion: An unsafe abortion is defined by WHO as a procedure for terminating an unintended pregnancy carried out by persons lacking the necessary skill and/ or in an environment that does not conform to minimum medical standards.

Introduction

The right to plan fertility was affirmed at the International Conference on Population and Development (ICPD) in Cairo, coordinated by the United Nations in 1994:

> All couples and individuals have the right to decide freely and responsibly the number and spacing of their children and to have access to the information and means to do so.
>
> (United Nations Population Fund, 1997)

The ICPD Conference was important in ratifying efforts to integrate reproductive and sexual rights issues into the agendas of international agencies such as the United Nations Population Fund (UNFPA) and the World Health Organization (WHO), and into the work of non-governmental organizations concerned with reproductive and sexual health. The action plans of governments on reproductive health now routinely include references to rights, sexuality, and gender equality in ways unimaginable before the ICPD. The prevention of unplanned pregnancy is crucial to the achievement of the Millennium Development Goals relating to the improvement of maternal health, the reduction of child mortality, and the eradication of poverty.

Meaning and measurement

A rich and growing body of research has helped to 'unpack' the concept of 'unplanned pregnancy'. Attempts to operationalize and measure it are essential to assessing the scale of the problem. Sources of confusion in the past have included the interchangeable use of terms like 'planned', 'intended' and 'wanted', and the uncritical application of the term 'unplanned' to pregnancies among younger women, for example, and those terminated, not all of which may be unplanned.

Activity 3.1

Methodological challenges beset efforts to measure unplanned pregnancy (Gipson et al., 2008). What might these be and how might they be addressed?

Feedback

- *People don't always think in dichotomous categories.* Few make a rigid distinction between planned and unplanned. The preference in research is increasingly to treat unplanned pregnancy not as a categorical variable (either/or), but as a continuous variable on a scale, accommodating a mid-way category representing 'ambivalence' (Bachrach and Newcomer, 1999). To some extent, any cut-offs are arbitrary, but they are useful provided they are well informed by common sense and science.
- *Assumptions of rationality may not be justified.* Expecting valid answers about planning status assumes greater awareness perhaps of motivation than most people

are privy to. Questions that tap several dimensions of the concept of 'planned' may be preferable to those eliciting 'yes/no' answers. Research is increasingly moving away from simply asking whether a pregnancy was intended or not, towards more sophisticated strategies using multi-item measures.

- *Perceptions of planning change over time.* A key question is whether hindsight reports are likely to provide accurate accounts of whether a pregnancy was unplanned. Most pregnancies – whether planned or not – become wanted, and this tendency increases with time from conception. So, too, does the tendency to describe them as intended, so that asking questions about planning status *after* the birth leads to a higher proportion being deemed planned than if asked during the pregnancy. Some studies have asked about planning status prospectively (Kavanaugh and Schwarz, 2009). The ideal would be to combine measures at different points in pregnancy and the postnatal period.

National surveys, such as the Demographic and Health Surveys (DHS), which provide data in most developing countries, elicit planning status using multidimensional questions probing intentions, contraceptive use, reactions to pregnancy and its timing, and desired family size. The US National Survey of Family Growth for many years set the standard for developed countries but its main focus was on fertility within marriage and most of the questions were developed before legal abortion was widely available.

In the early twenty-first century, a measure of unintended pregnancy was developed and tested among British women either seeking abortion or continuing a pregnancy (Barrett et al., 2004). Qualitative research carried out to inform design of the measure suggested that pregnancy planning involves: stopping contraceptive use; preparation for pregnancy (for example, making changes to diet and other health behaviours); timing in relation to life goals such as education and employment; contraceptive use; and discussion and agreement with a partner (Barrett and Wellings, 2002). These dimensions were incorporated into the measure alongside expressed intentions.

Prevalence and determinants of unplanned pregnancy

Of the 210 million pregnancies that occur annually worldwide, around 40% are estimated to be unintended (WHO, 2008). Of these, roughly equal proportions result in live births and abortions. In developed countries (where average desired family size is small), nearly half of the 28 million pregnancies that occur each year are assumed to be unplanned and, of these, those ending in abortion outnumber those resulting in live births by three to one. In developing countries (where average desired family size is still relatively large), just over a third of the 182 million pregnancies that occur each year are unplanned, and those resulting in live births outnumber those ending in abortion by five to four.

Prevalence of abortion

Over 90% of abortions result from unintended pregnancies (Lakha and Glasier, 2006). Data on abortions are routinely collected in most developed countries and are generally robust. In the developing world, reliable figures are less easily obtained and often refer only to married or cohabiting women. Data are less reliable in countries where abortion is restricted, since illegal abortions are not reported, and all abortions tend to be under-reported.

In 28% of the 193 countries in the world, abortion is permitted on request; in 34%, it is available on social or economic grounds. Elsewhere it is restricted, for example to cases where the mother's life is threatened by continuing pregnancy. In only four countries is abortion not permitted on any grounds (Malta, Vatican City, El Salvador, and Nicaragua). Recorded abortion rates vary little according to whether abortion is legal or not; the abortion rate is 29 per 1000 women of reproductive age in Africa where abortion is illegal in most countries and 28 per 1000 in Europe where it is mostly permitted on the most liberal grounds. Abortion rates are also surprisingly similar between developing and developed countries (26 and 29 per 1000 women of reproductive age, respectively). There are, however, marked variations between individual countries, from fewer than 10 per 1000 in the Netherlands, for example, to more than 50 per 1000 in Russia.

Factors associated with unplanned pregnancy

Marital status is the strongest predictor of unplanned pregnancy; the risk for single women is double that for married women. Younger age is also a risk factor, as is living in a rural area.

Social determinants play a major role in unintended pregnancy. A comparison of desired and actual family size shows that, almost universally, the burden of unintended pregnancy disproportionately falls on poorer women. In a study of poor women in New York City, 82% of pregnancies were unintended, compared with 49% for the United States as a whole (Besculides and Laraque, 2004). Poverty is compounded by gender inequality; the low status of women in many countries restricts their ability to make decisions relating to fertility. Having a larger family than is desired or affordable then perpetuates socio-economic and gender disparities.

Consequences of unplanned pregnancy

Birth outcomes

Unplanned pregnancy can have adverse health and economic outcomes for mothers and children, and for society at large (Marston and Cleland, 2003b; D'Angelo et al., 2004; Logan et al., 2007). These include less preparation for parenthood, failure or delay in uptake of prenatal care, and a higher risk of maternal morbidity and mortality. Some of these outcomes may relate to perceived social attitudes towards unplanned pregnancy; for example, women may be reluctant to present for antenatal care if they fear disapproval of their failure to control their fertility.

Unintended births have also been associated with higher rates of infant morbidity and mortality. Babies born as a result of unplanned pregnancies are of lower birth weight (possibly as a result of a greater likelihood of preterm delivery), are less likely to be breastfed, and have poorer mental and physical health during childhood. They reach lower levels of educational attainment and they grow up to be poorer. However, not all studies take into account factors such as poverty, which might have contributed to unplanned status initially.

Outcomes of abortion

Where abortion is illegal, it is usually unsafe (WHO, 2008). Legalization of abortion, such as in South Africa, and more recently Nepal, has resulted in a fall in the rate of unsafe abortions. Globally, roughly half of all abortions are unsafe and the vast majority of these are performed in the developing world. Unsafe abortion accounts for 13% of all maternal deaths. While in developed countries the mortality rate from abortion is less than one per 10,000 abortions, in Africa it is 65 per 10,000. Abortion complications are responsible for 72% of all deaths among Nigerian women aged under 19 (Raufu, 2002).

Unsafe abortions also cause substantial morbidity. In Egypt, the number of women hospitalized every year with abortion complications (216,000) is more than the total number of abortions performed annually in the UK (Singh, 2006). In developed countries, abortion is extremely safe – safer, for example, than it is to be sterilized and safer than having a baby.

Contraception and unplanned pregnancy

In theory, unplanned pregnancy – and hence its adverse consequences – should be preventable by use of contraception. An estimated 90% of abortion-related deaths and 20% of pregnancy-related deaths would be averted by effective contraception (Cleland et al., 2006b). In practice, the relationship between levels of contraceptive use and unintended pregnancy is complex. As use of contraception increases, we could expect abortion rates to fall. But the increased use of modern contraception in countries with high fertility rates usually coincides with a widespread desire for fewer children. Since contraceptive use is neither universal nor infallible, efforts to limit family size are associated with an increase in induced abortion (Marston and Cleland, 2003a).

Furthermore, as fertility rates decrease, the duration of exposure to the risk of unintended pregnancy increases. In the UK, where most couples have two children, and where average age at first sex is 16 years and that of the menopause is 51, most women spend more than 30 years trying to avoid pregnancy. No country to date has achieved low fertility levels without access to abortion.

Uptake of contraception

Until the twentieth century, efforts to limit family size were made largely by practising abstinence, infrequent sex, coitus interruptus (withdrawal), and breastfeeding. These methods were relatively successful: average family size declined in developed countries long before the advent of so-called modern contraceptives, and periodic abstinence, withdrawal, and lactational amenorrhoea continue to play a major role in some countries.

Today, patterns of contraceptive use vary worldwide both in terms of the prevalence of use of any method and of the types of methods chosen. The UN reports on patterns of use annually (United Nations, 2011). The proportion of married women of reproductive age (comparative rates for single women are not available) who used a method of contraception was 63% worldwide, 72% in the more developed regions, and 61% in the less developed regions. Rates of use also vary between developing countries. In Africa as a whole, 31% of women use contraception, but whereas in Kenya nearly half of married women do so, in Sierra Leone the figure is less than 10%. The reasons women in developing countries most commonly give for not using a method include concerns about health risks or side effects (23%), infrequent sex (21%), being postpartum or breastfeeding (17%), and opposition from partners (10%).

Contraceptive method use

Modern contraceptive methods are divided into reversible (hormonal, intrauterine, and barrier methods) and non-reversible (sterilization) methods. Despite a recent decline in uptake, female sterilization is still the most commonly used modern method of fertility control. One in five married couples relies on it and in Brazil, India and China, one in three. Vasectomy (male sterilization) is more popular in developed than in developing countries. Factors that have contributed to the decline in use of female sterilization include the availability of long-acting reversible methods of contraception (particularly the hormone-releasing intrauterine system), changes in service delivery, and demographic trends such as later childbearing and the increasing trend towards 'second families'.

The intrauterine device (IUD) is the world's most popular non-surgical method of contraception, largely because of its use by almost 36% of married women in China. However, the prevalence of use of intrauterine contraception varies widely between countries, with hardly any use in most African countries and the USA. Low uptake of intrauterine contraception in both developed and developing countries is attributed to misconceptions about the method, insufficient emphasis during contraceptive consultations, and insufficient provider experience.

The use of method is related to age and marital status (which are, of course, related to fertility intentions): younger women and single women are more likely to use the pill or male condom, while older women more likely to rely on sterilization or vasectomy. Hormonal contraception, particularly long-acting reversible contraceptive methods, could have a major impact on the reproductive health of young women in developing countries, but most rely on traditional methods such as withdrawal and natural family planning. While 37% of young, single women in Sub-Saharan Africa use contraception, only 8% use a hormonal method (Cleland et al., 2006a).

Among barrier methods, the male condom is by far the most commonly used and the only reversible method available for men. Despite the potential of condoms to reduce sensation and interrupt sex, and their association with disease in some contexts, easy access without the need for involvement of a health professional, together with absence of hormonal side effects and protection offered against sexually transmitted infections (STIs), offer advantages over other methods.

Incorrect/inconsistent use of contraception

Unplanned pregnancies result from not using contraception at all, and from not using it effectively. Researchers and clinicians distinguish between 'user failure' and 'method failure' (the method was used correctly, but did not work). The proportion of unplanned pregnancies that result from method failure is small, and varies with the method used (Figure 3.1).

Box 3.1 Methods of fertility control

Contraceptive sterilization: female or male. Use of female sterilization is in decline due to the availability of a choice of long-acting methods, changes in service delivery, and demographic trends such as later childbearing and more 'second families'.

Hormonal contraception: comprise *combined methods* containing both estrogen and progestogen and those containing *progestogen alone* (POC). Most commonly delivered as oral contraceptives, but combined preparations are also delivered via a transdermal patch, vaginal ring or a monthly injection; POC are available as injections (Depo Provera), implants, and the hormone-releasing intrauterine systems (see below).

Intrauterine contraceptives: the copper intrauterine device (IUD) provides up to 10 years of contraception. The main mode of action is to prevent fertilization, but if this occurs an IUD also inhibits implantation. The main side effect is menstrual change; periods are longer and may be more painful. The hormone-releasing intrauterine system (IUS) releases a tiny amount of progestogen daily and causes endometrial atrophy (thinning), which results in reduced menstrual bleeding.

Barrier methods: prevent sperm entering the upper female genital tract. The male condom is by far the most commonly used and the only reversible modern method available for men. Female condoms offer some protection against STIs, but diaphragms and cervical caps do not.

Spermicides: act by killing sperm. They are often used with other barrier methods to increase effectiveness. Spermicidal preparations containing nonoxynol-9 have an irritant effect on vaginal and penile tissue that may enhance the risk of HIV transmission.

Natural family planning: involves avoidance of intercourse during the fertile period of the cycle (periodic abstinence). The calendar (rhythm) method calculates the fertile period based on the length of the normal menstrual cycle. Others use hormone-related symptoms such as changes in cervico-vaginal mucus or a rise in basal body temperature (signifying that ovulation has occurred).

Breastfeeding: delays the resumption of fertility after childbirth, the length of the delay being related to the frequency and duration of breastfeeding and the timing of introduction of other food. Potential for use greater in countries in which women breastfeed for longer, and where modern methods of contraception are costly and difficult to obtain.

Emergency contraception: a drug or device used after intercourse to prevent pregnancy. Most hormonal emergency contraception preparations must be taken within 72 hours of intercourse, at most 5 days. All types work by preventing or delaying ovulation and not by interfering with implantation or causing an abortion. Copper IUD insertion is sometimes used as an alternative, especially if kept as an ongoing method. Emergency contraception prevents over 95% of pregnancies but if inserted after implantation will cause an abortion.

Induced abortion: a simple procedure, which, at early gestation (under 9 weeks), can be undertaken by nurses. It can be done surgically or by using drug regimens that induce miscarriage. The type of procedure is dictated by the gestation of the pregnancy, the availability of methods (drug regimes, particularly mifepristone, are legally restricted in places) and, in most developed countries, the woman's preference.

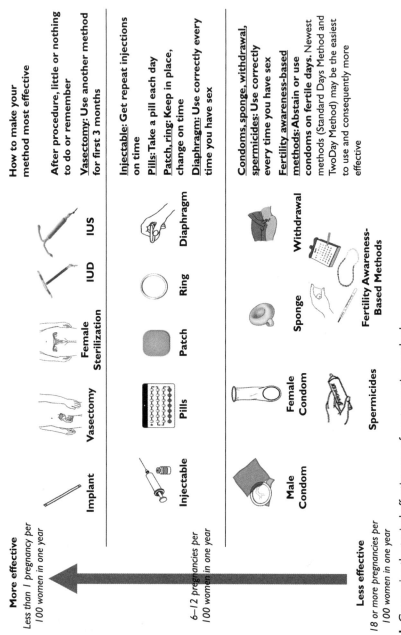

More effective
Less than 1 pregnancy per 100 women in one year

How to make your method most effective

After procedure, little or nothing to do or remember

Vasectomy: Use another method for first 3 months

Implant   Vasectomy   Female Sterilization   IUD   IUS

Injectable: Get repeat injections on time

Pills: Take a pill each day

Patch, ring: Keep in place, change on time

Diaphragm: Use correctly every time you have sex

6–12 pregnancies per 100 women in one year

Injectable   Pills   Patch   Ring   Diaphragm

Condoms, sponge, withdrawal, spermicides: Use correctly every time you have sex

Fertility awareness-based methods: Abstain or use condoms on fertile days. Newest methods (Standard Days Method and TwoDay Method) may be the easiest to use and consequently more effective

Male Condom   Female Condom   Spermicides   Sponge   Withdrawal   Fertility Awareness-Based Methods

Less effective
18 or more pregnancies per 100 women in one year

Figure 3.1 Comparing the typical effectiveness of contraceptive methods

Source: Trussell and Guthrie (2011)

Rates of user-failure also vary with the method. The scope for user failure of a contraceptive method depends on the mechanism of action, how easy it is to use, and the degree to which its use is independent of compliance. Methods such as intrauterine methods or implants, which once in place make no demands on the user, are the most effective; their typical-use failure rate is the same as that for perfect use. By contrast, user failure rates for natural methods of family planning are high, since many couples find it difficult to abstain from intercourse for the period required (up to 9 days). User failure rates are also high with methods of contraception, such as condoms, diaphragms, and withdrawal, that rely on correct use with every act of intercourse.

Compliance with contraceptives requiring daily action is demanding and may not be possible where people do not lead orderly lives. In a study in which women kept daily diaries and took their contraceptive pills from an electronic device that recorded use, 57% missed three or more pills every cycle and the average number missed in the third cycle of pill use was closer to six (Trussell, 2007). Because of the high prevalence of oral contraceptive use, poor compliance with oral contraceptives accounts for the majority of unplanned pregnancies.

Discontinuation of contraception

Discontinuation rates are higher for methods that do not require removal by a health professional, as is clear from Figure 3.1, which shows the percentage of couples in the USA still using each method at the end of one year. Young women in particular are likely to discontinue their contraceptive methods and up to 50% do so during the first three months of use.

Factors influencing uptake, choice, and continuation

Many factors determine whether a couple use contraception, which method is used and how effectively, and most are interlinked.

Availability and accessibility

How easily contraception can be obtained is fundamental in determining whether any method is used, and if so, which one. In an analysis of adoption of contraception in West Africa from 1991 to 2004, Cleland and colleagues (2011) reported access to contraceptives to be 'shockingly' limited.

In many societies, social disapproval of premarital sex limits young women's knowledge and access to health services. A systematic review of qualitative research examining the limits to modern contraceptive use by young women in five developing countries suggests that misconceptions are rife and services do little to dispel them (Williamson et al., 2009). The review quotes young women interviewed in a study in South Africa.

I take a pill when I know my boyfriend is coming and we probably going to make love. I sometimes forgot to take it before we make love so I take it after we made love.

There is nothing explained to us, it's just go through, what method do you want and if it's an injection they will inject you. The nurses always look busy and we are afraid to ask questions.

Patterns of contraceptive method use reflect social and cultural attitudes towards fertility control, sexuality, and the roles of women in society, together with the views of providers and promotion of certain brands of contraceptive by pharmaceutical companies. In Turkey, for example, empowerment of women in terms of better socio-economic status, better education, and more liberal attitudes towards women and family planning have coincided with reductions in use of withdrawal as the main method (Cindoglu et al., 2008).

Religious factors are important in determining contraceptive preferences in some contexts. The copper intrauterine device, for example, provides up to 10 years of contraception and is even safer than hormonal contraception, although cultural factors may militate against its use. Although its main mode of action is to prevent fertilization, it also reduces the likelihood of implantation if it occurs, of particular relevance in countries where Roman Catholicism predominates.

Acceptability

In the absence of a perfect contraceptive method, men and women are obliged to balance the costs and benefits of existing methods through the fertile period of their life based on a number of criteria. These include, in addition to availability and ease of access: how easy the method is to use, freedom from bothersome side effects, efficacy in preventing pregnancy, and actual and perceived safety – that is, absence of health risks.

These factors take on different importance through the reproductive life course. Among younger women who are not in regular relationships and who have not started a family, and for whom concerns about mortality are some way off, ease of use and efficacy may be valued more highly than freedom from health risks. At the stage of timing and spacing children, ease of use may be forfeited for freedom from concerns about the impact of contraception on fertility. In later life, as fertility declines, risk of adverse health outcomes may be prioritized over effectiveness.

Activity 3.2

The criteria governing method choice also vary culturally. Which side effects are seen as significant varies with the context in which the method is used. Thinking about your own cultural setting, which side effects do you think might be viewed as most significant?

Feedback

Most surveys of contraceptive use in developed countries highlight fear of weight gain as an important determinant of method choice. In a longitudinal survey of Swedish women, weight gain prompted one in five 19-year-old women to stop using the oral contraceptive pill (Larsson et al., 1997). By contrast, in a study of discontinuation of injectable contraceptive methods in six countries in Latin America, only four women in the study gave up for reasons relating to weight gain, compared with 23 who did so for bleeding-related reasons (Bassol et al., 2000).

Changed bleeding patterns (including amenorrhoea – no bleeding) are the most common reasons worldwide for discontinuation of hormonal methods. In some settings, heavier bleeding is seen as a problem. Qualitative research has shown that high discontinuation of IUD use among women in Bangladesh (half had given up within a year of insertion) is associated with increased menstrual bleeding. In Bangladesh, women cannot pray, have sexual intercourse, perform household tasks or participate in community activities during menstruation, and so heavy bleeding poses serious challenges to everyday life (Bradley et al., 2009).

In settings in which continued fertility is highly valued, lighter menstrual bleeding – or none at all – may be a problem. Where not being able to bear children poses a threat to social and economic survival, women like to be reassured of their fertility by the appearance of a monthly period (Williamson et al., 2009).

Interventions to reduce unintended pregnancy

Barriers to fertility regulation are an important determinant of the pace of fertility decline in many countries. Overcoming method-related reasons for contraceptive non-use could reduce unintended pregnancy by as much as 59%. The use of modern contraceptive methods has been successfully promoted for child spacing and limiting family size among older women with children in developing countries, but there is still considerable unmet need.

Increasing uptake of contraception requires action on a number of fronts, from improved access to clinical services and the broader range of contraceptive methods to changes in social norms. Negative perceptions relating to modern, reliable contraception methods need to be addressed, as do cultural norms and inaccurate beliefs around fertility. Understanding women's individual concerns and perspectives on family planning and contraceptive method use is important to efforts to encourage contraceptive uptake and continuation.

The demographic profile of non-users of contraception suggests that interventions to prevent unintended pregnancy should be tailored for the urban poor and should target unmarried, young women. In this sub-group, rates of non-use are high and the health consequences of unplanned pregnancy are of particular concern. Increasing uptake in this population sub-group requires the combined provision of information, life skills, support, and access to youth-friendly services. Since women who have one unintended pregnancy are more likely to have another, provision of family planning and contraceptive services as part of prenatal, postpartum, and post-abortion care can help reduce recurrence of unintended pregnancy.

Interventions aimed at improving contraceptive compliance at the individual level have proved disappointing. In China, sending women letters reminding them of their appointment for the injection combined with phoning them if they failed to attend had no effect on the number of appointments missed or continuation rates of Depo Provera® (Hou et al., 2010). And in the USA, daily SMS text messaging to remind women to take their pill had no effect on the number of pills missed (Trussell, 2007).

The use of emergency contraception has not been shown to reduce rates of unintended pregnancy or abortion at population level (Glasier et al., 2004). In part, this is because most women who could use it but do not are unaware of having been at risk of pregnancy. However, failure to use emergency contraception may also be due to fear of disapproval.

It is by now a cliché, but nevertheless a truism, that education is the best contraception. In both developing and developed countries, improvement in women's life, education, and employment chance is likely to be the strongest motivator to take up reliable methods of contraception.

Providing contraceptives and family planning services at low or no cost to the user helps to prevent unintended pregnancies. Subsidized family planning services improve the health of the population and save money for governments and health insurers by reducing medical, education, and other costs to society. Providing modern contraceptives to the 201 million women in developing countries who are at risk of unintended pregnancy and who do not have access to contraception would prevent an estimated 52 million unintended pregnancies annually. This would prevent 1.5 million maternal and child deaths annually, and reduce induced abortions by two-thirds.

Summary

Globally, unplanned pregnancy rates are high and have shown little sign of significant decline over recent decades. In many developed countries, the growing demand for smaller families, decreasing age at first sex (in some countries), and increasing age at marriage has meant that women spend much of their adult lives trying to avoid an unintended pregnancy. In some developing countries, lack of education and lack of access to effective methods contribute significantly to the problem.

Within and between countries, the burden of unintended pregnancy is not distributed equally but falls on poorer women, young women, and single women. Despite improvements in the lives of women generally, high rates of unintended pregnancy continue to impact negatively on women's lives, restrict their opportunities, and perpetuate the cycle of poverty.

With modern, highly effective contraceptives, the issue is less about method failure and more about access. In many areas, such methods are unavailable and/or unaffordable. Increasing use of long-acting reversible contraception (such as the IUD and contraceptive implants) decreases the chance of unintended pregnancy by decreasing the chance of incorrect use. The public health impact of reducing unplanned pregnancy in terms of narrowing social and health disparities, improving quality of life, and reducing maternal mortality rates would be considerable.

References

Bachrach CA and Newcomer S (1999) Forum: Intended pregnancies and unintended pregnancies: distinct categories or opposite ends of a continuum?, *Family Planning Perspectives*, 31(5): 251–2.

Barrett G and Wellings K (2002) What is a 'planned' pregnancy? Empirical data from a British study, *Social Science and Medicine*, 55(4): 545–57.

Barrett G, Smith SC and Wellings K (2004) Conceptualisation, development, and evaluation of a measure of unplanned pregnancy, *Journal of Epidemiology and Community Health*, 58(5): 426–33.

Bassol S, Cravioto MC, Durand M, Bailon R, Carranza S, Fugarolas J et al. (2000) Mesigyna® once-a-month combined injectable contraceptive: experience in Latin America, *Contraception*, 61(5): 309–16.

Besculides M and Laraque F (2004) Unintended pregnancy among the urban poor, *Journal of Urban Health*, 81(3): 340–8.

Bradley JE, Alam ME, Shabnam F and Beattie TS (2009) Blood, men and tears: keeping IUDs in place in Bangladesh, *Culture, Health and Sexuality*, 11(5): 543–58.

Cindoglu D, Sirkeci I and Sirkeci RF (2008) Determinants of choosing withdrawal over modern contraceptive methods in Turkey, *European Journal of Contraception and Reproductive Health Care*, 13(4): 412–21.

Cleland J, Ali MM and Shah I (2006a) Trends in protective behaviour among single vs. married young women in sub-Saharan Africa: the big picture, *Reproductive Health Matters*, 14: 17–22.

Cleland J, Bernstein S, Ezeh A, Faundes A, Glasier A and Innis J (2006b) Family planning: the unfinished agenda, *Lancet*, 368(9549): 1810–27.

Cleland JG, Ndugwa RP and Zulu ME (2011) Family planning in sub-Saharan Africa: progress or stagnation?, *Bulletin of the World Health Organization*, 89: 137–43.

D'Angelo DV, Gilbert BC, Rochat RW, Santelli JS and Herold JM (2004) Differences between mistimed and unwanted pregnancies among women who have live births, *Perspectives on Sexual and Reproductive Health*, 36(5): 192–7.

Gipson JD, Koenig MA and Hindin MJ (2008) The effects of unintended pregnancy on infant, child, and parental health: a review of the literature, *Studies in Family Planning*, 39(1): 18–38.

Glasier A, Fairhurst K, Wyke S, Ziebland S, Seaman P, Walker J et al. (2004) Advanced provision of emergency contraception does not reduce abortion rates, *Contraception*, 69(5): 361–6.

Hou MY, Hurwitz S, Kavanagh E, Fortin J and Goldberg AB (2010) Using daily text-message reminders to improve adherence with oral contraceptives: a randomized controlled trial, *Obstetrics and Gynecology*, 116: 633–40.

Kavanaugh ML and Schwarz EB (2009) Prospective assessment of pregnancy intentions using a single versus a multi-item measure, *Perspectives in Sexual and Reproductive Health*, 41(4): 238–43.

Lakha F and Glasier A (2006) Unintended pregnancy and use of emergency contraception among a large cohort of women attending for antenatal care or abortion in Scotland, *Lancet*, 368(9549): 1782–7.

Larsson G, Blohm F, Sundell G, Andersch B, Milsom I (1997) A longitudinal study of birth control and pregnancy outcome among women in a Swedish population, *Contraception*, 56(1): 9–16.

Logan C, Holcombe E, Manlove J and Ryan S (2007) *The Consequences of Unintended Childbearing: A White Paper*. Washington, DC: Child Trends, Inc. Available at: http://www.childtrends.org/Files/Child_Trends-2007_05_01_FR_Consequences.pdf.

Marston C and Cleland J. (2003a) Relationships between contraception and abortion: a review of the evidence, *International Family Planning Perspectives*, 29(1): 6–13.

Marston C and Cleland J (2003b) Do unintended pregnancies carried to term lead to adverse outcomes for mother and child? An assessment in five developing countries, *Population Studies*, 57(1): 77–93.

Raufu A (2002) Unsafe abortions cause 20,000 deaths a year in Nigeria, *British Medical Journal*, 325(7371): 988.

Singh S (2006) Hospital admissions resulting from unsafe abortion: estimates from 13 developing countries, *Lancet*, 368(9550): 1887–92.

Trussell J (2007) Contraceptive efficacy, in RA Hatcher, J Trussell, A Nelson, W Cates, F Stewart and D Kowal (eds.) *Contraceptive Technology*, 19th rev. edn. New York: Ardent Media.

United Nations, Department of Economic and Social Affairs, Population Division (2011) *World Contraceptive Use 2010* (POP/DB/CP/Rev2010). Available at: http://www.un.org/esa/population/publications/wcu2010/Main.html.

United Nations Population Fund (1997) *State of World Population 1997: The Right to Choose: Reproductive Rights and Reproductive Health.* New York: UNFPA. Available at: www.unfpa.org/swp/1997/swpmain. htm.

Williamson LM, Parkes A, Wight D, Petticrew P and Hart GJ (2009) Limits to modern contraceptive use among young women in developing countries: a systematic review of qualitative research, *Reproductive Health*, 6: 3.

World Health Organization (WHO) (2008) *Unsafe Abortion: Global and Regional Estimates of the Incidence of Unsafe Abortion and Associated Mortality in 2008*, 6th edn. Geneva: WHO.

Sexual violence

Claudia Garcia-Moreno,
Kirstin Mitchell and Kaye Wellings

Overview

In this chapter, we focus on sexual violence and its impact on health, including sexual health. We first clarify our terms and then provide an overview of the scale of the problem. We describe the behavioural and situational predictors of sexual violence, including the role of gender inequality, poverty, and conflict. Finally, we summarize the sexual health outcomes of the experience of sexual assault and examine possibilities for prevention.

Learning outcomes

After reading this chapter, you will be able to:

- Explain the concept of sexual violence
- Describe the scale of the problem globally and appreciate some of the challenges in measuring sexual violence
- Describe factors that increase the risk of sexual violence
- Identify the health consequences of sexual violence
- Discuss primary and secondary strategies for prevention

Key terms

Rape: Physically forced or otherwise coerced penetration – even if slight – of the vulva or anus, using a penis, other body parts or an object.

Sexual assault: Any form of assault involving a sexual organ, including coerced contact between the mouth and penis, vulva or anus.

Sexual violence: The WHO defines sexual violence as 'any sexual act, attempt to obtain a sexual act, unwanted sexual comments or advances, or acts to traffic, or otherwise directed, against a person's sexuality using coercion by any person regardless of their relationship to the victim, in any setting, including but not limited to home and work'.

Note: All definitions from Jewkes et al. (2002: 149).

Introduction

As noted in Chapter 1, a broadly based definition of sexual health includes the right to a satisfactory sexual life, free of violence and coercion. Sexual violence was recognized as a human rights problem by the United Nations relatively recently. It began to feature in international fora during the later decades of the twentieth century and public health policies were elaborated and ratified at the International Conference on Population and Development (ICPD) in Cairo in 1994 and at the World Conference on Women in Beijing in 1995.

Definitions

Definitions of sexual violence vary between and within countries. In the United States, for example, the Federal Bureau of Investigation defines rape as 'carnal knowledge' (vaginal intercourse) of a female forcibly and against her will, while the National Institute of Justice defines it as 'forced vaginal, oral or anal sex experienced by men or women'. Inclusion of oral or anal sex, and inclusion of men, in the second definition but not the first are both examples of common differences between definitions. Others include whether or not intimate partner or 'marital' rape feature in the formulation. But central to all definitions is the notion of coercion, however expressed.

Coercion covers a spectrum of force. Apart from physical force, it may involve intimidation, blackmail or threats, of physical harm or job loss, for example. It may occur when a person is unable to give consent, for instance, while drunk, drugged, asleep or otherwise incapable of understanding the situation (Jewkes et al., 2002). The range of acts related to sexuality that can involve coercion is also wide. It includes not only rape but forced marriage, forced pregnancy, female genital mutilation, sexual abuse of children, denial of the right to protect against pregnancy or a sexually transmitted infection (STI), forced prostitution, and trafficking of people for the purpose of sexual exploitation (Jewkes et al., 2002). While sexual violence can take these many forms, the focus of this chapter is on rape, defined above under the key terms.

Estimating and measuring prevalence

Before the landmark studies of sexual violence carried out by Mary Koss in the United States, little academic research had been undertaken to measure its prevalence. The setting up of rape crisis centres in the USA in the early 1970s, however, revealed the widespread extent of sexual assault in American society and provided the impetus for further investigation. Koss and colleagues found that one in four US college women had experienced rape in their lifetime and 84% knew their attacker (Koss et al., 1987). Rape was not scarce, and it was not primarily a 'stranger-in-the-bushes' phenomenon. It was a violent crime committed against millions of women by men they knew (Campbell and Wasco, 2005: 128).

Most sexual violence is committed by men and most men are known to the women they rape. The US National Survey found that 43% of all rapes reported were by a current or former intimate partner, and only 17% were by a stranger (Tjaden and Thoennes, 2000). In a study of 11 European countries (Lovett and Kelly, 2009), two-thirds of perpetrators were known to their victim and one in four were current or former partners.

Studies carried out into sexual violence have shown no sign of a decline in prevalence (Campbell and Wasco, 2005). They also show that throughout the world, sexual violence is more common than is often supposed. Comparative data were, until recently, derived from reviews of national studies of sexual violence. These studies estimated the proportion of women forced to have sex at some time in their lives at between 10% and 30% (Tjaden and Thoennes, 2000; Stacey and Falik, 2001; Watts and Zimmerman, 2002).

In 2003, the WHO Multi-country Study on Women's Health and Domestic Violence was launched using a common methodology, and provided more robust comparative data on several dimensions of violence (Garcia-Moreno, 2005). This cross-national study of sexual violence is a population-based household survey of over 24,000 women aged 15–49 years, involving 15 sites in 10 countries (Bangladesh, Brazil, Ethiopia, Japan, Namibia, Peru, Samoa, Serbia and Montenegro, Thailand, and Tanzania). The proportion of women reporting their first experience of sexual intercourse to have been unwanted ranged from 3% to 30%, and the proportion of women reporting their first sexual encounter as forced ranged between 3% and 24%. In Bangladesh, Ethiopia, Peru province, and Tanzania, over 14% of women reported that their first sexual experience was forced.

Estimates of lifetime prevalence of sexual violence by an intimate partner ranged from 6% of women in Japan to 59% in Ethiopia (Figure 4.1) (Garcia-Moreno, 2005). Reports by women of sexual violence after the age of 15 by men who were not intimate partners varied from fewer than 1% in Ethiopia and Bangladesh (where it is not uncommon for women to be married by 15 years) to 10–12% in Peru, Samoa, and urban Tanzania (Garcia-Moreno, 2005).

Sexual violence against men

Sexual violence against men is under-reported. The stigma and shame attached to it appear even stronger than in the case of women. Sexual violence against men may be particularly prevalent in male-dominated settings such as prisons. Sexual violence against men is being increasingly documented in situations of armed conflict. The problem is under-researched but what data exist suggest that in developing countries, the number of men who have been sexually assaulted ranges from 3.6% (Namibia) to around 20% (Peru) (WHO, 2002).

Perpetration of sexual violence

Recently, researchers have asked men about their perpetration of sexual violence against women. In a household study of over 1500 randomly selected men aged 18–49 years in South Africa, 28% reported having raped a woman and 5% had done so in the previous 12 months (Jewkes et al., 2011). Of those men reporting that they had raped someone, three-quarters reported first doing so before they were 20 and more than half had raped on more than one occasion. These reported rates are within the range of experiences of sexual assault reported by women across the world (Garcia-Moreno, 2005).

Challenges in measuring prevalence

The data from different studies show a good deal of variability in the prevalence of sexual violence. This may represent real differences in the experience of sexual violence

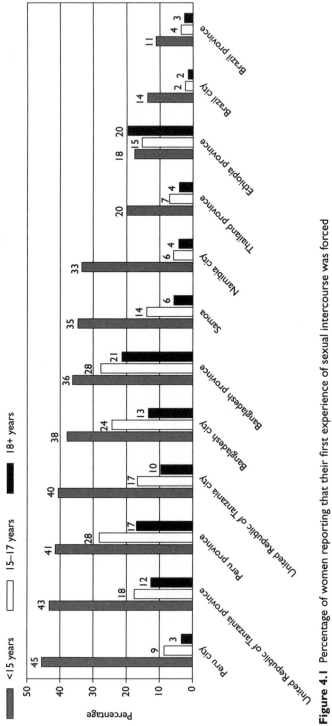

Figure 4.1 Percentage of women reporting that their first experience of sexual intercourse was forced

Note: Japan city, Serbia and Montenegro city, and Thailand city are not represented because of the low percentages reporting first sex before the age of 15 years

Source: WHO (2005: 14)

in different cultural contexts, or it may reflect research effects, including the source of the data, the characteristics of the sample, the definition of violence used, and differences between settings and across time in willingness to report.

Source of the data

Prevalence data are drawn from a variety of sources, including routinely kept police records and health service statistics, as well as community surveys. Estimates of the scale of sexual violence derived from routine statistics are less reliable than those based on survey data. Routine statistics from police records and health service statistics are not only lower bound estimates but may also be biased.

Activity 4.1

Why do you think routine statistics might underestimate the problem?

Feedback

Rape is often not reported to the police and not everyone who experiences it seeks medical help. Women may be reluctant to report for a number of reasons: they may fear disapproval and/or disbelief; they may feel shame at their experience; or they may see attempts to do so as futile because of inadequate support systems. Police or health service records also under-represent rape by an intimate partner. In contexts in which social norms oblige a wife to meet her husband's sexual demands, many women may not report marital rape as sexual assault and may not seek health care.

Surveys represent the method of choice in assessing the scale of the problem, but operationalizing the concept of sexual violence is challenging. The way in which questions are posed impacts significantly on disclosure (Koss, 1992). It is now widely agreed that asking questions about specific behavioural acts produces more accurate estimates. Because questions describe exactly the behaviour being asked about, respondents are cued to recall more accurately what they have experienced. This is preferable to general questions about 'being raped', for example, which are open to individual and cultural variations in interpretation.

The WHO Multi-country Study operationalized intimate partner sexual violence using the following three questions:

- Were you physically forced to have sexual intercourse when you did not want to?
- Did you have sexual intercourse when you did not want to because you were afraid of what your partner might do?
- Were you forced to do something sexual that you found degrading or humiliating?

For non-partner sexual violence, the question was:

- Since the age of 15 years has anyone (other than your partner/husband) ever forced you to have sex or to perform a sexual act when you did not want to?

Activity 4.2

How do you think definitions and wording of questions might influence reporting of sexual violence?

Feedback

Broad definitions that include a wide range of behaviours are likely to lead to higher rates of reporting.

Wording of questions is particularly important when asking about behaviours that are seen as shameful or censured by society. Respondents may not be able to admit to 'rape' but might be willing to admit to 'coercing' another person into sex. In this context, a slightly leading question would be acceptable to overcome the bias towards non-reporting. For instance, 'How many times have you forced a woman ...' rather than 'Have you forced a woman ...'.

Risk factors associated with sexual violence

Understanding why some people perpetrate sexual violence, and why others become victims of it, is essential to the design of effective interventions.

Factors associated with experiencing sexual violence

The risk of sexual violence is greater for younger men and women, and the earlier sexual intercourse occurs, the higher the likelihood that it is forced. Adults with a history of abuse during childhood (Mangioloi, 2009) or who have previously been raped are more likely to be raped again. Other risk factors include poverty, harmful drug and alcohol use, being involved in sex work, having many sexual partners, homelessness, and mental and physical disability (WHO, 2002; Tavara, 2006).

Factors associated with perpetration of sexual violence

Men who rape are more likely themselves to have been raped by a man, or to have been subjected to abuse as a child. They are also more likely to have had limited education and to have experienced adversity as a child. Problem or heavy drinking has also been shown to be a strong predictor of rape perpetration (Tsai et al., 2011). A family environment characterized by violence, few resources, strong patriarchy, and a lack of emotional support is also a key risk factor (WHO, 2002). Perpetrating rape is also associated with less equitable views on gender relations; in the South African study by Jewkes et al. (2011), the most common motivation reported was sexual entitlement (the belief that a husband is entitled to have sex with his wife when he wants to). Another common motive is to demonstrate power or to punish the victim for a moral transgression (WHO, 2002).

Social contextual factors

The research focus is often on individual-level risk factors for sexual violence, to the neglect of risk factors associated with the social context. In fact, social norms can create an environment that is supportive of sexual violence, thereby increasing prevalence. Such social norms include those which condone violence against women, support male superiority and inequitable relationships, and endorse male entitlement to sex (for example, the belief that sex is a man's right, that men cannot control their sexual urges, and that rape is a sign of masculinity). Such attitudes can sometimes be found among those professionally tasked with supporting women who are victims of sexual violence. A study in Hong Kong revealed that one in three doctors working in an emergency department believed responsibility for preventing rape rested with the woman (Wong et al., 2002).

Weak community and legal sanctions also increase the likelihood of rape. Although rape is criminalized in most countries, it frequently goes unpunished. In many cultures, marriage is seen as granting privilege with regard to sex, and marital rape is not recognized in the law. Such practices create an environment in which rape can be perpetrated with impunity. Women may be deterred from seeking justice for fear of not being believed, or even of being punished. In some countries (Egypt, for example), the victim may even be killed to restore 'family honour' (WHO, 2002).

Rape is common in conflict situations as a tactic of war or ethnic cleansing. Its use as a weapon against the enemy is documented in a number of settings, including Timor, Sudan, Bosnia, Algeria, and the Congo (Chelala, 1998; Watts and Zimmerman, 2002; Hynes et al., 2004; Johnson et al., 2010). Exposure to sexual violence during civil war in the Democratic Republic of the Congo was reported by 18% of women after the war (Casey et al., 2011). Soldiers may rape women and girls to brutalize and humiliate the perceived 'enemy'. Men, too, may be raped, or forced to witness the rape of their female relatives. The Platform for Action adopted at the Fourth World Conference on Women in Beijing in 1995 declared rape in armed conflict to be a war crime and under certain circumstances to be considered genocide. Sexual violence also occurs as a result of general disorganization and the normalization of violence (Wood, 2006). It is common in refugee or internally displaced people's camps.

The risk factors for experiencing and perpetrating both sexual violence and intimate partner violence are summarized in Table 4.1.

Health effects of sexual violence

Sexual violence has major health, behavioural, and social consequences, both short and long term.

Activity 4.3

Note down what you think may be possible consequences of sexual violence.

Feedback

Compare your list with the consequences discussed in the following paragraphs.

Table 4.1 Risk factors for sexual violence and intimate partner violence (adapted from WHO/LSHTM, 2010)

Level of influence	Men perpetrating violence	Women experiencing violence
Individual		
Demographic	Low income and educational level	Young age; low education; separated or divorced
Childhood experiences	Experience of sexual abuse; witness to parental violence	Witness to parental violence
Mental illness	Antisocial personality	Depression
Substance use	Harmful use of alcohol and illegal drugs	Harmful use of alcohol and illegal drugs
Attitude towards violence	Acceptance of violence	Acceptance of violence
Relationship	Multiple partners/infidelity; low ability to resist pressure from peers	
Community	Poverty; ineffective sanctions within community	Poverty; ineffective sanctions within community
Societal	Social and gender norms that condone violence	Social and gender norms that condone violence

Sexual violence has serious consequences for health and these can be both physical and psychological in nature. They may include physical injuries and, in extreme cases, death. Psychological consequences include depression, social phobias, anxiety, and even attempted suicide (Rees et al., 2011). Rape trauma syndrome describes a cluster of common reactions that disrupt everyday functioning. In addition to the psychological consequences just described reactions may include, among others, difficulty sleeping and eating, withdrawal from friends, family and activities, and a sense of helplessness. Difficulty adjusting to normal life after rape may lead to further risk behaviour, including harmful drug and alcohol use (Hegarty et al., 2004) as well as sexual risk-taking.

The risk of acquiring an STI as a result of a single act of rape is estimated at between 4% and 30% (Kawsar et al., 2004). The level of risk depends on the baseline level of STIs within the community as well as the risk associated with the individual perpetrator. The risk of acquiring HIV during a sexual assault is usually lower, but increases where injury to the genital area allows a direct portal of entry for the virus. Even where no infection has occurred, the fear that it might have can increase the emotional trauma associated with rape. Studies also show an elevated lifetime risk of STIs, including HIV, for women who have experienced sexual violence.

The risk of pregnancy following a single experience of rape is no greater than from that resulting from consensual unprotected sex. But since pregnancies following rape are virtually all unwanted, many end in abortion and in countries with restrictive abortion laws, many of these are unsafe abortions. Even in countries in which the law permits abortion following rape, there may be medical and administrative barriers to termination of pregnancy.

The experience of sexual assault can have lasting effects on sexual and reproductive functioning. Women who have been raped may develop a fear of sex or may experience sexual function problems, such as loss of desire and lubrication difficulties (Steel and

Herlitz, 2007). They are more likely than women who have not been raped to experience gynaecological complaints such as endometriosis, menstrual irregularities, and chronic pelvic pain (Weaver, 2009). Physical effects are not limited to sexual health; women who have been sexually assaulted are more likely to report several chronic diseases, somatic symptoms, and functional limitations (Golding, 1994).

The physical and psychological health consequences experienced by men are similar to those of women but men may be particularly concerned for their masculinity, and may fear others think they are homosexual or powerlessness to prevent rape. Among adolescent boys, studies show a link between experiencing rape and troubled behaviour, such as stealing, absenteeism from school, violence, and drug abuse (WHO, 2002).

The social consequences of sexual violence can also be severe; victims may be stigmatized and shunned by their families and community (WHO, 2002). In the long term, the experience of sexual assault can affect educational and employment chances, emotional wellbeing, and quality of life. Qualitative research in the Democratic Republic of the Congo shows consequences of conflict-related rape far beyond the physiological and psychological trauma associated with the attack, including community isolation and shame not only among victims but also their partners and family members (Kelly et al., 2012).

Prevention

Despite its high prevalence and serious consequences, sexual violence is rarely included as a component of sexual and reproductive health programmes. Primary prevention strategies include changing social norms and attitudes that condone violence and foster ideas of masculinity based on male superiority and sexual entitlement, as well as laws that discriminate against women. Creating a climate of no tolerance is important and needs to include national legislation and supportive policies to ensure equal rights for women to education, work, and social security, the ability to enter or leave a marriage freely and to have equal property rights.

Targeting men as perpetrators is a promising approach, but identifying effective interventions with this aim is not easy. Early prevention, which focuses on minimizing exposure to trauma during childhood, is an important element (Jewkes et al., 2011). Some programmes aimed at reducing aggressive behaviour and re-educating male perpetrators of sexual assault have been found to have lasting effects (Garrity, 2011). There has been less consideration of how prevention initiatives can shift social perceptions of blame for rape from victims to perpetrators (Suarez and Gadalla, 2010). Programmes such as 'Stepping Stones', developed in Africa to address issues such as gendered relations, have been effective at getting community members to discuss the issue of violence within a more comprehensive programme of peer workshops. Such approaches show promise in bringing about norm change. In some places, men themselves have formed community action groups to campaign against sexual violence, such as the 'Men Can Stop Rape' group in Washington, DC (WHO, 2002).

Programmes delivered in schools to prevent dating violence, such as Safe Dates in the United States (Foshee et al., 2004) and Fourth R in Canada (Wolfe et al., 2009), have been shown to have some effect in reducing dating violence, and adaptations of some of these curricula are now being tested in South Africa.

At the level of secondary prevention, provision of comprehensive post-rape care services is critical. In the short term, survivors of rape need compassionate care and psychological first aid. They also require emergency contraception and information on safe abortion, STI treatment and prophylaxis, HIV prophylaxis when appropriate, and quality forensic examination (if a woman decides to pursue prosecution). Immediate mental health support (such as firmly reassuring the woman that she is not to blame) can impact on later recovery. In the USA and Canada, sexual assault nurse examiner (SANE) programmes, in which specially trained forensic nurses provide 24-hour first-response care to sexual assault victims, have been shown to have positive effects on emotional recovery (Ahrens et al., 2000).

Pleas have been made for clinical care for sexual assault victims to be integrated into primary health care. However, lack of awareness of the signs and symptoms of sexual violence and how to identify it often militates against provision of adequate prevention and care. Opportunities for detection may also be limited by women's reluctance to be examined. A substantial minority of women object to routine questions about sexual violence (Cold et al., 2004).

Building awareness and knowledge of sexual violence among health providers, police, and the justice sector is necessary, as is improving the implementation of existing laws and reforming them where necessary to ensure they service the needs of survivors. Advances have been made in recent years, especially in terms of justice for victims of rape and healthcare provision. In health care, advances in some contexts include more widespread use of standard protocols and 'sexual assault evidence kits'. In terms of justice, advances in some countries has included improvements to the efficiency of processing cases, broadening the legal definition of rape, providing legal aid to victims, and the introduction of minimum sentencing (WHO, 2002). For further progress to be made, a multidisciplinary strategy is needed involving multiple sectors, including education, health, social support, police, and criminal justice.

Summary

Women are more likely to be the victims of rape than men, and they are more likely to be raped by someone they know than by a stranger. Sexual violence merits greater public health attention than it currently receives for several reasons: it involves a serious violation of human rights, it is common and it is not becoming less so, and it has severe and often long-lasting consequences for mental and physical health.

An effective public health response to sexual violence requires intervention at several levels. Primary prevention should address social norms condoning sexual violence against women, particularly within intimate relationships, and should seek to convince both perpetrator and victim that blame attaches to the former. In terms of secondary prevention, increasing awareness and knowledge of sexual violence among health providers is necessary, as is addressing the longer-term health and social consequences.

Disclaimer

Claudia Garcia-Moreno is a staff member of the World Health Organization. The authors alone are responsible for the views expressed in this publication and they do not necessarily represent the decisions, policy or views of the World Health Organization.

References

Ahrens CE, Campbell R, Wasco SM, Aponte G, Grubstein L and Davidson WS (2000) Sexual assault nurse examiner (SANE) programs: an alternative approach to medical service delivery for rape victims, *Journal of Interpersonal Violence*, 15: 921–43.

Campbell R and Wasco SM (2005) Understanding rape and sexual assault: 20 years of progress and future directions, *Journal of Interpersonal Violence*, 20: 127–31.

Casey SE, Gallagher MC, Makanda BR, Meyers JL, Vinas MC and Austin J (2011) Care-seeking behavior by survivors of sexual assault in the Democratic Republic of the Congo, *American Journal of Public Health*, 101(6): 1054–5.

Chelala C (1998) Algerian abortion controversy highlights rape of war victims, *Lancet*, 351(9113): 1413–14.

Cold J, Petruckevitch A, Cheng WS, Richardson J, Moorey S, Cotter S et al. (2004) Sexual violence against adult women primary care attenders in east London, *British Journal of General Practice*, 54: 135–6.

Foshee VA, Bauman KE, Ennett ST, Linder GF, Benefield T and Suchindran C (2004) Assessing the long-term effects of the Safe Dates program and a booster in preventing and reducing adolescent dating violence victimization and perpetration, *American Journal of Public Health*, 94(4): 619–24.

Garcia-Moreno C (coordinator) (2005) *WHO Multi-country Study on Women's Health and Domestic Violence Against Women*. Geneva: WHO.

Garcia-Moreno C, Jansen H, Ellsberg M, Heise L and Watts C, on behalf of the WHO Multi-country Study on Women's Health and Domestic Violence against Women Study Team (2006) Prevalence of intimate partner violence: findings from the WHO multi-country study on women's health and domestic violence. *The Lancet*, 368(9543): 1260–1269.

Garrity SE (2011) Sexual assault prevention programs for college-aged men: a critical evaluation, *Journal of Forensic Nursing*, 7(1): 40–8.

Golding J (1994) Sexual assault history and physical health in randomly selected Los Angeles women, *Health Psychology*, 13(2): 130–8.

Hegarty K, Jun J, Chondros P and Small R (2004) Association between depression and abuse by partners of women attending general practice: descriptive, cross-sectional survey, *British Medical Journal*, 328: 621–4.

Hynes M, Robertson K, Ward J and Crouse C (2004) A determination of the prevalence of gender-based violence among conflict-affected populations in East Timor, *Disasters*, 28: 294–321.

Jewkes R, Sen P and Garcia-Moreno C (2002) Sexual violence, in E Krug, L Dahlberg, JA Mercy, AB Zwi and R Lozano (eds.) *World Report on Violence and Health*. Geneva: WHO.

Jewkes R, Sikweyiya Y, Morrell R and Dunkle K (2011) Gender inequitable masculinity and sexuality entitlement in rape perpetration South Africa: findings of a cross-sectional study, *PLoS One*, 6(12): e29590.

Johnson K, Scott J, Rughita B, Kisielewski M, Asher J, Ong R et al. (2010) Association of sexual violence and human rights violations with physical and mental health in territories of the Eastern Democratic Republic of the Congo, *Journal of the American Medical Association*, 304(5): 553–62.

Kawsar M, Anfield A, Walters E, McCabe S and Forster GE (2004) Prevalence of sexually transmitted infections and mental health needs of female child and adolescent survivors of rape and sexual assault attending a specialist clinic, *Sexually Transmitted Infections*, 80: 138–41.

Kelly J, Kabanga J, Cragin W, Alcayna-Stevens L, Haider S and Vanrooyen MJ (2012) 'If your husband doesn't humiliate you, other people won't': gendered attitudes towards sexual violence in eastern Democratic Republic of Congo, *Global Public Health*, 7(3): 285–98.

Koss MP (1992) The underdetection of rape: methodological choices influence incidence estimates, *Journal of Social Issues*, 48(1): 61–75.

Koss MP, Gidycz CA and Wisniewski N (1987) The scope of rape: incidence and prevalence of sexual aggression and victimization in a national sample of higher education students, *Journal of Consulting and Clinical Psychology*, 55: 162–70.

Lovett J and Kelly L (2009) *Different Systems, Similar Outcomes? Tracking Attrition in Reported Rape Cases in 11 European Countries*. London: Child and Women Abuse Studies Unit, London Metropolitan University. Available at: http://www.cwasu.org/publication_display.asp?pageid=PAPERS&type1&pagekey=44&year=2009 (accessed 24 October 2011).

Mangioloi R (2009) The impact of child sexual abuse on health: a systematic review of reviews, *Clinical Psychology Review*, 29(7): 647–57.

Rees S, Silove D, Ivancic L, Steel Z, Creamer M, Teesson M et al. (2011) Lifetime prevalence of gender-based violence in women and the relationship with mental disorders and psychosocial function, *Journal of the American Medical Association*, 306(5): 513–21.

Stacey P and Falik M (2001) Prevalence of violence and its implications for women's health, *Women's Health Issues*, 11: 244–58.

Steel JL and Herlitz CA (2007) Risk of sexual dysfunction in a randomly selected nonclinical sample of the Swedish population, *Obstetrics and Gynecology*, 109(3): 663–8.

Suarez E and Gadalla TM (2010) Stop blaming the victim: a meta-analysis on rape myths, *Journal of Interpersonal Violence*, 25(11): 2010–35.

Tavara T (2006) Sexual violence, *Best Practice and Research in Clinical Obstetrics and Gynaecology*, 20(3): 395–408.

Tjaden P and Thoennes N (2000) *Full Report of the Prevalence, Incidence and Consequences of Violence Against Women: Findings from the National Violence Against Women Survey*. Report NIJ 183781. Washington, DC: National Institute of Justice.

Tsai AC, Leiter K, Heisler M, Iacopino V, Wolfe W, Shannon K et al. (2011) Prevalence and correlates of forced sex perpetration and victimization in Botswana and Swaziland, *American Journal of Public Health*, 101(6): 1068–74.

Watts C and Zimmerman C (2002) Violence against women: global scope and magnitude, *Lancet*, 359(9313): 1232–7.

Weaver TL (2009) Impact of rape on female sexuality: review of selected literature, *Clinical Obstetrics and Gynecology*, 52(4): 702–11.

Wolfe DA, Crooks C, Jaffe P, Chiodo D, Hughes R, Ellis W et al. (2009) A school-based program to prevent adolescent dating violence: a cluster randomized trial, *Archives of Paediatrics and Adolescent Medicine*, 163(8): 692–9.

Wong AY, Wong TW, Lau PF, Lau CC (2002) Attitude towards rape among doctors working in the emergency department, *European Journal of Emergency Medicine*, 9(2): 123–6.

Wood K (2006) Sexual violence in developing countries, in R Ingham and P Aggleton (eds.) *Promoting Young People's Sexual Health: International Perspectives*. Abingdon: Routledge.

World Health Organization (WHO) (2002) *World Report on Violence and Health*. Geneva: WHO.

World Health Organization (WHO) (2005) *WHO Multi-country Study on Women's Health and Domestic Violence against Women. Summary Report – Initial Results on Prevalence, Health Outcomes and Women's Responses*. Geneva: WHO.

World Health Organization (WHO) (2010) *Preventing Intimate Partner and Sexual Violence Against Women: Taking Action and Generating Evidence*. Geneva: WHO.

Sexual function, pleasure, and satisfaction

Kirstin Mitchell

Overview

Sexual activity is a fundamental human pleasure. When sexual function problems interfere with the experience of pleasure, it can be distressing for both the individual and their partner. In this chapter we explore what it means to experience sexual function, pleasure, and satisfaction. We then describe the main sexual function problems, examines their causes and consequences, and explore issues surrounding diagnosis, measurement, and treatment. Finally, we consider some public health approaches to promoting sexual wellbeing.

Learning outcomes

After reading this chapter, you will be able to:

- Explain what is meant by sexual function, pleasure, and satisfaction
- Assess different perspectives with regard to understanding sexual function
- Describe the challenges involved in defining and measuring sexual function problems
- Identify the most common problems and their causes
- Explain the need for public health interventions to promote sexual function, pleasure, and satisfaction, in particular those that adopt a psychosocial as well as biomedical approach

Key terms

Sexual function: The ability to participate in a sexual relationship as one would wish. This is the converse of the WHO definition of sexual dysfunction: 'The various ways in which an individual is unable to participate in a sexual relationship as he or she would wish. Sexual response is a psychosomatic process and both psychological and somatic processes are usually involved' (WHO, 1994).

Sexual response: A psychosomatic response (genital, cognitive, physiological, and emotional) to an erotic stimulus (such as being touched by a partner) leading to a change in subjective state.

Introducing sexual function

In Chapter 1, we learned that the WHO definition of sexual health concerns physical, emotional, mental, and social wellbeing in relation to sexuality, as well as the possibility of pleasure (WHO, 2006). According to this definition, sexual function – the ability to participate in a sexual relationship as one would wish – is central to the fulfilment of sexual health. Conversely, problems with sexual function can cause significant psychological morbidity both for individuals and their partners. Yet within the public health sphere, sexual function problems are often overlooked as a component of sexual health, particularly in developing countries facing more urgent priorities (such as HIV/AIDS) and in culturally conservative countries where discussion of sexual pleasure is difficult.

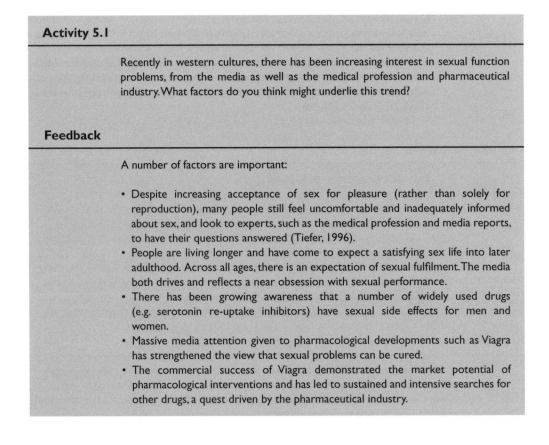

Activity 5.1

Recently in western cultures, there has been increasing interest in sexual function problems, from the media as well as the medical profession and pharmaceutical industry. What factors do you think might underlie this trend?

Feedback

A number of factors are important:

• Despite increasing acceptance of sex for pleasure (rather than solely for reproduction), many people still feel uncomfortable and inadequately informed about sex, and look to experts, such as the medical profession and media reports, to have their questions answered (Tiefer, 1996).
• People are living longer and have come to expect a satisfying sex life into later adulthood. Across all ages, there is an expectation of sexual fulfilment. The media both drives and reflects a near obsession with sexual performance.
• There has been growing awareness that a number of widely used drugs (e.g. serotonin re-uptake inhibitors) have sexual side effects for men and women.
• Massive media attention given to pharmacological developments such as Viagra has strengthened the view that sexual problems can be cured.
• The commercial success of Viagra demonstrated the market potential of pharmacological interventions and has led to sustained and intensive searches for other drugs, a quest driven by the pharmaceutical industry.

Introducing pleasure and satisfaction

Sexual satisfaction has been defined as 'an affective response arising from one's subjective evaluation of the positive and negative dimensions associated with one's sexual relationship' (Lawrance and Byers, 1995: 268). Sexual pleasure, though more focused on activity, is also relative, and is often as much a product of expectation, of the symbolic meaning of the act (Tiefer, 2004), and of the emotional and relational context as it is of the physical experience.

A historical perspective

Social attitudes towards the expression of sexual pleasure and gratification tend to be characterized at best by ambivalence, and at worst by shame, fear, and disgust. This is partly the legacy of religious traditions that viewed the body (and carnal pleasures) as an impediment to achieving purity of the soul (an idea introduced by Plato). Bodily pleasures came to be seen as sinful and in need of tight control (Dening, 1996). Not all religions have viewed sex negatively; ancient Eastern religions such as Taoism and Tantric Buddhism saw spirituality and sensuality as harmonious, and viewed sex as a way of exploring spirituality (Dening, 1996). Such ideas enabled greater freedom of sexual expression and gave fewer reasons for guilt and shame.

In most societies throughout history, patriarchal control of women's sexual behaviour has limited their ability to freely experience pleasure (Dening, 1996). They have been viewed either as lustful beings whose voracious appetites require strict control (as in ancient Hebrew times) or as frigid and sexually passive (Dening, 1996). In Victorian England, the physician Dr. William Acton once declared that 'the majority of women (happily for them) are not very much troubled with sexual feeling of any kind' (Acton, 1867: 144). To an extent, this view is still evident today in the sexual double standard that maintains that men should be sexually active while women should be sexually chaste.

Understanding variation in sexual response

Sex is fundamental to procreation, and positive sexual expression is often central to intimate relationships. That said, it is important to be aware that there is great variation in sexual response (Chapter 1) and some people live long and satisfying lives without having sex (Bancroft, 2009).

Masters and Johnson (1966) were the first to investigate patterns of sexual response at the individual and physiological level. They used laboratory observations to describe four distinct temporal phases characteristic of heterosexual intercourse: excitement or arousal, plateau phase, orgasm, and resolution. Known as the human sexual response cycle (HSRC), their model gave rise to a three-stage derivative model of desire, arousal, and orgasm that became the basis for contemporary medical understanding of sexual dysfunction. Although Masters and Johnson provided a major service in showing that women were as capable of experiencing as much sexual pleasure as men, their work on the HSRC has been criticized by Tiefer and others, who point out that in their efforts to reveal universal physiological patterns of sexual behaviour in laboratory conditions, they failed to take account of real-life variation in sexual response (Tiefer, 1996).

The influence of different perspectives

Recent research into sexual function problems has in large part been dominated by the biomedical perspective, which focuses on physiological responses, particularly genital function. However, a significant minority of professionals working in the field have a psychosocial perspective, which focuses on the psychological, relational, and social aspects of sexual encounters. They criticize the biomedical perspective, arguing that it separates body from mind, that it assumes a universal sexual body independent of social and relational influences, and that it reduces sexuality to the physical function of the genitals (biological reductionism) (Tiefer, 1996). In particular, the biomedical perspective is less good at explaining female sexuality because, as Bancroft (2002) asserts:

* vaginal intercourse often fails to meet women's sexual needs;
* the sexual responses of females are more variable than those of males and are often best understood as adaptations to circumstance; and
* female sexuality is more prone to influence by social and cultural constraints.

Our understanding of sexual function has been shaped by thought systems (such as medicine and religion), social movements (notably feminism), and historical events (such as the introduction of Viagra). All definitions of sexual function problems need to be seen as products of their time. There are many examples of sexual disorders that have disappeared from the clinical textbooks when later shifts in thinking have exposed them as unfounded and possibly harmful. For instance, Freud's insistence that clitoral orgasms were psychically immature led many women who were unable to achieve vaginal orgasms to be diagnosed with a psychiatric condition called 'frigidity'.

A contemporary concern for some is the increasing influence of the pharmaceutical industry on research into sexual function problems.

Activity 5.2

Why do you think the influence of the pharmaceutical industry might be of concern?

Feedback

* The focus of the pharmaceutical industry on biomedical intervention underplays the influence of complex psychological, relational, political, and socio-cultural factors (Tiefer, 2000).
* The ethos of secrecy and profit conflicts with scientific openness and thus potentially hampers progress in the field (Tiefer, 2000).
* Finally, the profit motive encourages the industry to expand the potential market as far as possible, leading to an over-emphasis on the severity of problems and inflated estimates of the number of people thought to experience problems (Moynihan et al., 2002). This is known as 'disease mongering', which includes 'broadening the definitions of diseases in such a way as to include the greatest number of people' (Payer, 1992: 54). Experiences that fail to meet some normative standard for sexual activity become pathologized (e.g. women who do not have 'enough' sexual desire or men who ejaculate 'too early').

A global view

Much more is known about sexual function problems in the USA and Europe than elsewhere. This is because the field is dominated by western research. In non-western societies, sexual function problems tend to attract much less attention and funding.

Activity 5.3

What factors do you think influence the level of awareness about sexual function problems within individual countries?

Feedback

- The amount of exposure to western culture and media, as well as the strength of traditional and/or religious conservatism, will affect the degree of openness about sexual matters in general and sexual function problems in particular.
- Access to information is important. This may be determined by the country's level of development (e.g. number of literate people with access to the Internet) as well as the extent to which the government controls access to information.
- The status of women in society will influence the extent to which female sexual concerns (beyond fertility) are regarded as legitimate. The level of gender equality may also influence the extent to which women can raise these issues with their partners.
- Without adequate service provision, there may be a perception that no effective treatment exists, and there may seem little point in even talking about one's problems.
- Lack of service provision may be due to a country having more urgent sexual health priorities, such as HIV/AIDS.

What data exist suggest that sexual function problems vary across cultures, and that some of this variance can be attributed to differences in cultural attitudes towards, and beliefs about, sexual activity. For instance, Dhat syndrome (anxiety about losing semen accompanied by somatic symptoms such as fatigue) is prevalent almost exclusively in Oriental cultures. The origins of the syndrome may be traceable to traditional belief systems (Ayurvedic and Taoist) which place immense importance on semen and which stress the importance of not wasting it. And, for instance, in rural China, where over a third of rural couples report little or no foreplay, 37% of wives report painful sex (Francoeur and Noonan, 2004).

In countries such as Nigeria, where fertility is a key indicator of a functioning sex life, concerns with erectile function predominate (Francoeur and Noonan, 2004). East Asian students in the USA are said to report lower sexual desire than their Caucasian peers, a finding that has been partly explained by differences in levels of conservatism and guilt about sex (Woo et al., 2010). Many psychosocial factors associated with sexual function vary by culture. These include the level of gender equality, the acceptability of expressing feelings and emotions, and the adequacy of sex education.

Defining and classifying sexual function problems

Sexual dysfunction concerns the physical, emotional, and psychosocial functioning of a sexual relationship. The term 'dysfunction' implies that part of the sexual response system is malfunctioning. Diagnosis of sexual dysfunction requires a clinical history to assess the severity of symptoms and rule out physical or psychological causes. The term 'sexual function problems' can be used to describe self-reported problems where no clinical history has been taken.

Classification of sexual function problems

The diagnosis and measurement of sexual dysfunction is usually based upon the International Classification of Diseases (ICD-10) (WHO, 1994) and the Diagnostic and Statistical Manual of Mental Disorders (DSM-IV TR) of the American Psychiatric Association (2000). An abridged version of ICD-10 is shown in Box 5.1 and gives an idea of the different types of problems that individuals and couples experience.

Box 5.1 Abridged version of the classification of sexual dysfunction in ICD-10 (WHO, 1994)

Lack or loss of sexual desire
- Loss of desire is principal problem
- Lack of desire does not preclude enjoyment but makes initiation less likely

Sexual aversion and lack of sexual enjoyment
- Prospect of sexual interaction is associated with strong negative feelings
- Fear and anxiety lead to avoidance of sexual activity
- Lack of sexual enjoyment
- Normal sexual response but lack of appropriate pleasure

Failure of genital response
- Men – difficulty in developing or maintaining an erection suitable for satisfactory intercourse
- Women – vaginal dryness/failure of lubrication

Orgasmic dysfunction
- Orgasm does not occur or is markedly delayed
- May be situational or invariable

Premature ejaculation (men)
- Inability to control ejaculation sufficiently for both partners to enjoy sexual interaction

Non-organic vaginismus (women)
- Spasm of the muscles surrounding the vagina, causing occlusion of vaginal opening
- Penile entry either impossible or painful

Non-organic dyspareunia
- Pain during sexual intercourse
- Only used if no other primary sexual dysfunction and no pathological condition
- Occurs in men and women

Excessive sexual drive
- Only diagnosed if not secondary to an affective disorder

Other sexual dysfunction, not caused by organic disorder or disease
Unspecified sexual dysfunction, not caused by organic disorder or disease

---

The ICD-10 and DSM-IV TR classifications of sexual dysfunction, though widely used, are not universally accepted. One criticism is that sexual behaviour occurs predominately in couples but the classification systems focus only on individuals. A second – and major – criticism concerns the fact that these systems have limited clinical usefulness because patients often present for clinical help with a range of overlapping problems. Finally, these classifications do not adequately capture real-life variety across individuals, couples, and cultures. For example, in parts of the central Democratic Republic of Congo, a dry vagina is reportedly associated with increased pleasure and a wet (well-lubricated) vagina is seen as problematic (Brown et al., 1993).

How common are sexual function problems?

Table 5.1 summarizes prevalence figures for different sexual problems, using data from NATSAL 2000 (Mercer et al., 2003) and the Australian Study of Health and Relationships (ASHR) (Richters et al., 2003).

Table 5.1 Reported prevalence of different sexual function problems in Britain and Australia

	NATSAL				ASHR	
	≥1 month		≥6 months		≥1 month	
	M	F	M	F	M	F
n = *	4888	4826	4877	4818	8517	8280
Lacked interest in having sex	17.1	40.6	1.8	10.2	24.9	54.8
Were unable to come to a climax ψ	5.3	14.4	0.7	3.7	6.3	28.6
Came to a climax too quickly ψ	11.7	1.3	2.9	0.2	23.8	11.7
Experienced pain during intercourse	1.7	11.8	0.3	3.4	2.4	20.3
Did not find sex pleasurable	—	—	—	—	5.6	27.3
Felt anxious about performance	9.0	6.7	1.8	1.5	16.0	17.0
Had trouble achieving or maintaining an erection (men)	5.8	—	0.8	—	9.5	—
Had trouble lubricating (women)	—	9.2	—	2.6	—	23.9
At least one of the above problems	34.8	53.8	6.2	15.6	46.5	70.9

* Samples are weighted ψ or 'experience an orgasm'.

Source: Abridged from Bancroft (2009). Reproduced with permission.

Activity 5.4

Using Table 5.1, identify the most and least common problem among men and women. What strikes you as noteworthy about this table?

Feedback

- 'Lack of interest' is the most common problem reported by women. Among men, the short-term problem most commonly reported is lack of interest, but the persistent problem (lasting 6 months or more) most commonly reported is coming 'to a climax too quickly'.
- 'Experiencing pain' is the least common problem reported by men and coming 'to a climax too quickly' is the least common problem reported by women.
- The prevalence of problems is significantly higher in the Australian study compared with the British one. This probably results from differences in study design or sample. The mean age of participants was higher in the Australian than the British study and a different question format may have been used.
- The prevalence of reported problems decreases significantly where questions are about persistent rather than short-term problems.

A challenge of community surveys is that of collecting sufficiently detailed information to differentiate actual function problems (as clinically defined) from transient or adaptive changes in behaviour. This is harder to do for women than men, partly because what researchers define as problematic does not always correspond to what women see as such. A British study of 400 women attending their primary healthcare service found that one in five women felt they had no sexual dysfunction yet were defined by the researchers as having so, and a similar proportion felt they had sexual dysfunction but were defined by the researchers as not having so (King et al., 2007).

Activity 5.5

Despite decades of research, there is no standard way of measuring sexual function in the community. In what ways do you think the lack of standardization might cause problems?

Feedback

Lack of standardized measurement limits comparison of prevalence rates across studies and leads to uncertainty as to the 'true' burden of ill health. One study compared results from four different self-report instruments used within the same questionnaire and found that each produced a different prevalence estimate of sexual function problems among the women participants (Hayes et al., 2008).

The evidence is that men and women seek clinical help for different sexual problems. Men predominantly attend services for problems associated with genital response (most commonly erectile difficulties, followed by premature ejaculation), women for lack of interest and enjoyment, followed by vaginismus and painful sex (Bancroft, 2009).

The relational nature of sexual function problems

Relationship factors – the sexual partner as well as the interaction between partners – are often fundamental to the causes and experience of sexual difficulties. For women in particular, sexual and relationship problems are often interlinked. A British study showed that between half and two-thirds of women thought that difficulties with their partner lay at the base of their sexual problems (King et al., 2007). Co-morbidity of sexual problems in partners is common; in around one-third of patients with sexual dysfunction, the partner also has dysfunction (Gregoire, 1999); and when one partner receives individual therapy for a sexual problem, there is often also improvement in sexual functioning for the other partner (Gregoire, 1999).

Causes of sexual function problems

In addition to relational factors, Tiefer and colleagues (as part of their 'New View' campaign (http://fsd-alert.org)) identified three categories of factors that can cause sexual function problems: (1) sociocultural, political or economic factors (such as inadequate sex education, fear of judgement or punishment by cultural community or religious institutions, and lack of interest, fatigue and time due to work or family obligations); (2) psychological factors (such as guilt, shame, as well as the effects of depression or anxiety); and (3) physiological or medical factors (medical conditions, e.g. affecting the neurological or vascular systems, pregnancy and sexually transmitted infections, side effects of medical treatments). Usually, several different factors contribute to the experience of problems.

The public health impact of sexual function problems

The public health impact of sexual function problems has received very little attention. This may in part be attributed to the difficulty of accurately assessing the burden of disease. Measurement is challenging because of the difficulty of identifying universally applicable principles. Expectations and priorities vary by age and gender, as well as across cultures. In societies where female pleasure is not viewed as a legitimate concern, for instance, women may accept lack of orgasm or painful sex as 'normal'. Another issue is that even in countries where services exist, few of those reporting problems to surveys actually seek professional help (Mercer et al., 2003). Thus any estimate of the public health burden is likely to be an underestimate. Finally, it is often difficult to disentangle cause and effect. For instance, depression and poor sexual function are associated but the relationship is likely to be bi-directional.

Regardless of the direction of causality, sexual function problems are associated with significant psychological morbidity (including anxiety and loss of self-esteem) as well as relationship difficulties (possibly leading to break-up with negative consequences for individuals and families). Distress relating to sexual function problems is common, particularly among younger people. It may be caused by feelings of failure, shame, and anxiety, as well as frustration at not being able to experience pleasure. Sexual function problems can be distressing to couples trying to conceive, particularly in societies in which fertility is viewed as the key indicator of female sexual response. And where sexual dissatisfaction leads one or both partners to go outside the relationship, there is an increased risk of sexually transmitted infections and unplanned pregnancy.

Public health interventions

In contemporary western society, interventions are overwhelmingly targeted at individuals and focused on pharmacological treatment. The trend towards biomedical intervention has been driven in large part by the pharmaceutical industry, and is shored up by a well-meaning medical profession, anxious to provide patients with the quick fixes they request. Although PDE5 inhibitors such as Viagra have been widely regarded as a panacea, their side effects are not insignificant. They are unsuitable for men with certain pre-existing health conditions, and they are not always appreciated by the men's female partners. In general, medical and surgical intervention is unlikely to solve problems stemming from a complex array of psychological and relational issues. While acknowledging the benefits for some individuals, public health interventions need to look beyond ensuring the availability of medical and surgical treatment.

At a population level, public health interventions can do much to challenge norms in beliefs, attitudes, and behaviours that contribute towards negative experiences of sex. However, addressing norms is tricky. A particular challenge is to avoid being swayed by the politics and morality of the day. For example, where masturbation was condemned by some members of the British medical profession throughout much of the eighteenth and nineteenth centuries, today it is sometimes recommended as a treatment for premature ejaculation and orgasm dysfunction.

A starting point for public health interventions is to address ignorance and misinformation. In cultures where discussion of sexual matters is restricted, interventions may need to provide basic information, such as about the connection between inadequate foreplay and painful sex for women. In cultures already barraged by 'information' about sex, interventions could tackle unrealistic expectations about performance and promote a model of sex that is simply good enough, that does not necessarily hinge on vaginal penetration as the only route to pleasure, and that acknowledges more than one script for sexual function (Mitchell et al., 2011).

An obvious (though difficult) route for norm change is via sex education for school children and youth. The ideal would be an education that allows young people to explore some of the historical myths about sexuality, to explore how sex and sexuality are socially constructed in their society, to seriously critique the sexual double standard, and to discuss freely issues such as guilt and pleasure. As we discuss in Chapter 13, the inclusion of these topics is likely to be met with political resistance in most settings.

Other avenues for intervention are education campaigns targeting health professionals, and better provision of integrated services that combine both pharmacological and psychosocial approaches. More broadly based interventions that promote empowerment for women or which tackle other aspects of sexual health, such as sexual violence, childhood abuse, and availability of contraception, are likely to impact on sexual function as an indirect result.

Summary

Sexual function problems prevent an individual from participating in a sexual relationship as he or she would wish by interfering with the experience of pleasure. Our understanding of sexual function has been dominated by a western biomedical perspective, influenced by the pharmaceutical industry. This perspective tends to focus on genital function and tends to negate variation in sexual response, and variations in cultural expectations of sex. It is difficult to measure the public health impact of sexual function problems because of lack of agreement about how to define and measure them, as well as difficulty untangling the direction of cause and effect. Public health interventions need to look beyond ensuring the availability of medical and surgical treatment. They need to challenge norms in beliefs, attitudes, and behaviours that contribute to negative experiences of sex.

References

Acton W (1867) *The Functions and Disorders of the Reproductive Organs in Childhood, Youth, Adult Age, and Advanced Life, Considered in Their Physiological, Social, and Moral Relations*. Philadelphia, PA: Lindsay & Blakiston.

American Psychiatric Association (APA) (2000) *Diagnostic and Statistical Manual of Mental Disorders*, 4th edn. (DSM-IV TR). Washington, DC: APA.

Bancroft J (2002) The medicalisation of female sexual dysfunction: the need for caution, *Archives of Sexual Behaviour*, 31: 451–5.

Bancroft J (2009) *Human Sexuality and its Problems*. London: Elsevier.

Brown J, Ayowa OB and Brown RC (1993) Dry and tight: sexual practices and potential AIDS risks in Zaire, *Social Science and Medicine*, 37(8): 939–94.

Dening S (1996) *The Mythology of Sex: An Illustrated Exploration of Sexual Customs and Practices from Ancient Times to the Present*. London: Batsford.

Francoeur RT and Noonan RJ (eds.) (2004) *Continuum Complete International Encyclopedia of Sexuality*. New York: Continuum.

Gregoire A (1999) Assessing and managing male sexual problems, in J Tomlinson (ed.) *ABC of Sexual Health*. London: BMJ Books.

Hayes RD, Dennerstein L, Bennett C and Fairley CK (2008) What is the 'true' prevalence of female sexual dysfunctions and does the way we assess these conditions have an impact?, *Journal of Sexual Medicine*, 5: 777–87.

King M, Holt V and Nazareth I (2007) Women's views of their sexual difficulties: agreement and disagreement with clinical diagnosis, *Archives of Sexual Behavior*, 36: 281–8.

Lawrance K and Byers ES (1995) Sexual satisfaction in long-term heterosexual relationships: the interpersonal exchange model of sexual satisfaction, *Personal Relationships*, 2: 267–85.

Masters WH and Johnson VE (1966) *Human Sexual Response*. London: Churchill.

Mercer CH, Fenton KA, Johnson AM, Wellings K, Macdowall W, McManus S et al. (2003) Sexual function problems and help seeking behaviour in Britain: national probability sample survey, *British Medical Journal*, 327(7412): 426–7.

Mitchell K, Wellings K, King M, Nazareth I, Mercer C and Johnson A (2011) Scripting sexual function, *Sociology of Health and Illness*, 33(4): 540–53.

Moynihan R, Heath I and Henry D (2002) Selling sickness: the pharmaceutical industry and disease mongering, *British Medical Journal*, 324(7342): 886–91.

Payer L (1992) *Disease-mongers: How Doctors, Drug Companies and Insurers are Making You Feel Sick*. New York: Wiley.

Richters J, Grulich AE, de Visser RO, Smith AMA and Rissel CE (2003) Sexual difficulties in a representative sample of adults, *Australian and New Zealand Journal of Public Health*, 27: 164–70.

Tiefer L (1996) The medicalisation of sexuality: conceptual, normative and professional issues, *Annual Review of Sex Research*, 7: 252–82.

Tiefer L (2000) Sexology and the pharmaceutical industry: the threat of co-optation, *Journal of Sex Research*, 37(3): 273–83.

Tiefer L (2004) *Sex is not a Natural Act and Other Essays*. Boulder, CO: Westview Press.

Woo JS, Brotto LA and Gorzalka BB (2010) The role of sex guilt in the relationship between culture and women's sexual desire, *Archives of Sexual Behaviour*, 40: 385–94.

World Health Organization (1994) *ICD-10: International Statistical Classification of Diseases and Related Health Problems*, 10th edn. Geneva: WHO.

World Health Organization (2006) *Defining Sexual Health*. Report of a Technical Consultation on Sexual Health. Geneva: WHO.

PART 3

Risk and vulnerability

Young people

Kirstin Mitchell, Kaye Wellings and Maria Zuurmond

Overview

Young men and women under 25 represent over half the world's population and shoulder a significant portion of the burden of sexual ill health. In this chapter, we outline the basis for treating them as a target group for sexual health interventions. We examine patterns and trends in young people's sexual behaviour and we explore the influences on these. Finally, we identify priorities for intervention to protect young people's sexual health.

Learning outcomes

After reading this chapter, you will be able to:

- Explain why a sexual health focus on young people is important
- Describe patterns and trends in the sexual behaviour of young people
- Identify some of the influences on the sexual behaviour of young people
- Explain why young people are more vulnerable and often at greater risk, and recognize which young people may be at increased risk
- Assess priorities for intervention to improve the sexual health of young people

Key terms

Menarche: Onset of menstruation.

Young people: Men and women in the transition between childhood and adulthood, broadly aged 10–24 years.

What do we mean by young people?

The focus in this chapter is on the transitional period between childhood and adulthood. The length of this period varies greatly across cultures; in some it may last 20 years, in others less than one. A number of terms are used to describe people at this time of life, including adolescents, teenagers, youth, and young people but they tend not to be applied consistently. Several criteria are used to define this category, not only age, but also single status, degree of independence and, in some contexts, education. Age is clearly the most important qualifier but there is little agreement even on that.

The UK Department of Health variously defines young people as aged 16–19, under 20, and 16–25.

The term 'adolescence', from the Latin *adolescere*, to 'grow up', is in widespread use in this context. Social aspects are included in many instances of its use, but it tends to denote a fairly fixed maturational phase characterized by rapid physical and mental development. Like the term 'teenager', it is widely applied to the age group 10–19 years. Use of the term 'young people', by contrast, has the merit of admitting the variability in what constitutes a 'young person', in different cultures and at different times. It also acknowledges that young people may continue to be at heightened risk of adverse sexual health outcomes until way into their twenties. For this reason, we use the term 'young people' throughout this book.

Young people may be seen both as a risk group and an audience group in respect of their sexual health needs and opportunities:

- As a *risk group*: a reading of Chapters 2–5 shows that being young is a risk factor for a range of sexual health outcomes, including coercive sex, unplanned pregnancy, and sexually transmitted infections (STIs). This period of life is characterized by experimentation and risk-taking, such that even equipped with knowledge and skills, young people sometimes opt not to minimize risk. Young people may also be more vulnerable because of their lower position within social hierarchies, and their lack of power, control, and autonomy relative to adults. This can make it difficult for them to refuse unwanted sexual advances, to practise safer and satisfying sex, and to seek sexual health services.
- As an *audience group*: at this stage of life, attitudes and behaviours are not set in stone. The period of transition to adulthood represents a window of opportunity for shaping risk behaviour. Knowledge and skills gained early in life equip young people to critically appraise the myriad and conflicting messages they receive about sexuality, from medical sources ('sex carries risk of disease and pregnancy'), moral agendas ('unmarried sex is wrong'), and the media ('sex is exciting and reputation enhancing').

Activity 6.1

How do you think young people and adults might differ in the way they assess risks associated with sexual behaviour?

Feedback

Young people often assess risks of sexual behaviour differently to adults, seeing immediate benefits to sex in terms of developing autonomy, creating an identity, and acquiring kudos. They also tend to discount longer-term consequences, for example, infertility arising from STIs. Adults (including parents and public health professionals) and young people do not always agree on what counts as a problem. Whereas adults focus on health risks, young people may be more concerned about risks to their reputation and social standing. So whereas an adult might view early motherhood as a problem, a young woman might view it as offering status and emancipation from her parental home.

Onset of sexual activity

The early sexual behaviour of young people involves a variety of practices that do not necessarily culminate in intercourse. Nevertheless, the occasion of first sexual intercourse is seen as an important milestone and is an event of immense social and personal significance. The event has major health implications, since it marks initiation into the sexual act, which, if unprotected, carries the highest risk of such adverse outcomes as unplanned pregnancy and STIs. The status of virginity, which is still of great cultural and legal importance, is technically defined in terms of experience of sexual intercourse.

In only a small and diminishing number of societies does the age of biological sexual maturity coincide with the age deemed socially acceptable for sexual activity. This disjuncture between biological readiness for sexual activity and the socially approved timing of its expression underlies many of the problems relating to the maintenance of sexual health of young people. A balance has constantly to be sought between helping young people to safeguard their sexual health by providing the necessary information and resources with which they can avoid unplanned pregnancy and STIs and, at the same time, avoiding appearing to encourage premature sexual activity.

Activity 6.2

Public interest and research have tended to focus on the timing of first sexual intercourse. How do you think the criteria used to judge whether the timing is appropriate might have changed over the last half century?

Feedback

The ways in which timing of first sex has been construed have changed over time.

Half a century ago, the terms used to describe inappropriate timing were in relation to its occurrence in or out of marriage. In the 1960s and 1970s, the term 'premarital sex' dominated the literature relating to sexual behaviour of young people in developed countries. In societies in which early marriage is the norm and sex before marriage is less socially accepted, it still does. This reflects an assumption that first experience of sexual intercourse should occur within marriage (Biddlecom et al., 2008).

By the end of the twentieth century, the preoccupation had shifted to the age at which first intercourse should ideally occur. Words used in the literature, like 'early' and 'premature', reflect normative assumptions in this respect. What age is considered 'early' depends to some extent on the complexity of the society. In many societies, young people are expected to delay sexual relationships until they have completed the increasingly lengthy process of induction into adult life. In countries in which there is a law of sexual consent, this also tends to determine the age before which sexual debut is considered inappropriate. In developed countries, this is generally 16, in developing countries 15.

Today, public health researchers have begun to see criteria such as age and marital status as too crude to be used as the sole arbiters of when sexual activity should begin. Neither age nor marital status reliably safeguard sexual health status (Brown et al., 2001; Wight and Henderson, 2004). Adverse sexual health outcomes of first sex occur independently of age at the time. And in some countries in South Asia and sub-Saharan Africa, where early marriage is encouraged to protect young women's honour, sexual experiences can be coercive and traumatic and early pregnancy may be dangerous for mother and child. Young married women may find themselves powerless within their relationship and isolated from social support (UNICEF, 2011).

Increasingly, it is acknowledged that what is needed is a concept of timing that takes account of the wide personal and cultural variation in what is considered appropriate. Attempts are being made to think in terms of minimum requirements that should be in place for first sex to be seen as safe and satisfying (Wellings et al., 2001).

Activity 6.3

What criteria do you think are most important in defining first sex as safe and satisfying?

Feedback

The researchers who carried out the British National Study of Sexual Attitudes and Lifestyles made an assumption that first intercourse should, ideally, be:

- *Consensual* (both partners equally willing)
- *Protected* (contraception was used)
- *Timing not regretted* (its occurrence was considered not too soon or too late)
- *Autonomously decided* (not influenced by peer pressure or being drunk or high).

These four variables were used to construct a measure of 'sexual competence' at first sex (Wellings et al., 2001). The NATSAL researchers found a close fit between age at first sex and sexual competence defined in this way. But it was not a perfect fit. Ninety-one percent of women and 67% of men who reported first intercourse at 13 or 14 years were categorized as not sexually competent, but so too were 30% of those who had sex when they were 18 or older (Wellings et al., 2001). Lack of competence at first sex was found to be associated with having an abortion before 18, with subsequently having an STI, and with later sexual difficulties. These associations persisted even after taking age at first sex into account (Wellings et al., 2001).

Few studies have reported on pleasure or enjoyment at the time of first sexual intercourse. Those that have done so have shown that fewer than half of young people assessed their first sexual experience positively (Wight et al., 2008), and negative experiences were characterized by less control and planning, both of which are predictors of worse sexual health outcomes. Furthermore, research shows that many young people do not regard the timing of their first sexual experience to have been ideal. A third of young women considered intercourse to have occurred too soon, and the figure rose to 50% if they were under 16 at the time (Wellings et al., 2001). Retrospective data, however, need to be interpreted with caution. Reported feelings about a decision made some time ago may reflect present-day views and what happened subsequently. For a sizeable minority of young people, first sexual intercourse occurs against their will, and the harms associated with this are as yet relatively uncharted (see Chapter 4).

Patterns and trends in young people's sexual behaviour

Globally, sexual activity begins for most young people between the ages of 15 and 19 years but there is substantial variation between men and women and across regions. In most societies, young people have traditionally been expected to delay sex and childbearing until they have completed the increasingly lengthy process of induction into adult life. In general, and in line with the longer period of time spent in education, age at first sexual activity begins later in more developed countries than it does in those that are less developed.

In the richer countries of the world, however, first sexual intercourse is now experienced earlier than in previous decades (Wellings et al., 2006). In Europe, North America, and Australasia, for example, age at first sex dropped dramatically in the second half of the twentieth century, a trend that coincided with a relaxation on norms governing sex before marriage, increasing autonomy of young people, and access to birth control. Data from Britain (Wellings et al., 2001) show median age at first intercourse to have dropped by 5 years for women (from 21 to 16) and by 4 years for men (from 20 to 16) during this period, a dramatic social change and one that has important policy implications.

In countries in which first sexual intercourse most commonly occurs within marriage, such as in South Asia and in most parts of Africa, the trend has been in the opposite direction. As age at marriage has increased, so too has age at first sex. This is less true of young men, for whom age at first intercourse is not linked to age at marriage. Where premarital sex is more common among men than women, men are more likely to report having sex with sex workers (Brown et al., 2001).

The proportion of unmarried young people having sex varies widely across countries (Figure 6.1). In some, as in Azerbaijan and the Republic of Georgia for example, less than 1% of unmarried 15- to 19-year-olds have had intercourse (Bearinger et al., 2007). In contrast, fewer than 1% of young people in Britain today have their first experience of sexual intercourse within marriage, compared with two-thirds half a century ago.

The gap between age at first sex and settling with a live-in partner is considered a higher-risk period because of the potential for sexual experimentation and more transitory partnerships. As age at marriage increases and the period spent in full time education lengthens, this gap widens. There are large differences between the sexes and wide variation across areas with respect to these transitions (Figure 6.2).

Sexual partnerships and practices

Much is made of the supposed increase in sexual activity among young people. In many parts of the world today, young people are likely to have larger numbers of sexual partners than did their parents' generation. Nevertheless, the dominant lifestyle pattern among the young is one of serial monogamy rather than concurrent partnerships. The majority of young people in their teenage years report one or no sexual

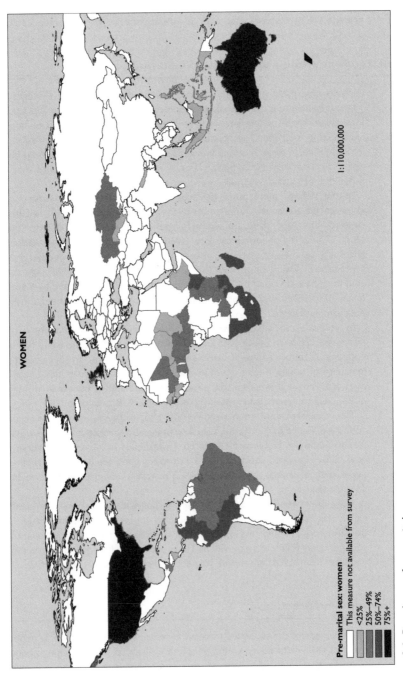

WOMEN

Pre-marital sex: women
☐ This measure not available from survey
☐ <25%
☐ 25%–49%
▨ 50%–74%
■ 75%+

1:110,000,000

Figure 6.1 Prevalence of premarital sex: women

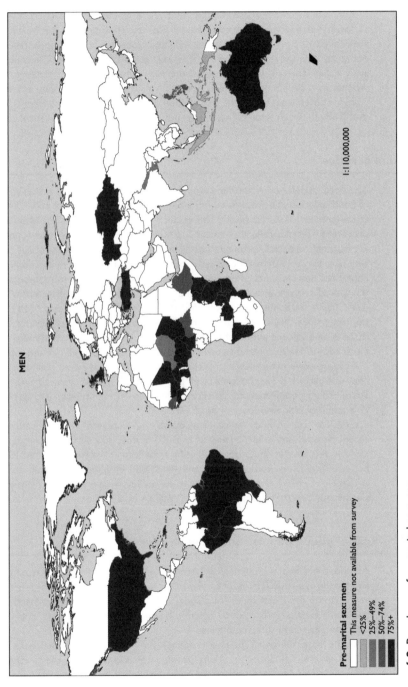

MEN

Pre-marital sex: men

This measure not available from survey

<25%

25%–49%

50%–74%

75%+

1:110,000,000

Figure 6.2 Prevalence of premarital sex: men

partners in a given year and, generally speaking, single people have sex less frequently than do their married counterparts (Wellings et al., 2006).

Again the differences between the sexes are often marked. In western-style democracies, in which women have achieved considerable success in gaining equality in other areas of life, the proportion of young men and women reporting more than one partner today is roughly equal. However, this was not always the case. These countries have seen a shift towards a narrowing of the gap in sexual behavior between men and women in recent times. But in countries in which women have not achieved equal status in other areas of life, the sexual double standard persists and there is still a gender divide between what is and what is not permissible in terms of sexual conduct.

Risk reduction practice

The need to delay pregnancy and avoid infection among the young makes the practice of contraception and prophylaxis (disease prevention) an important public health focus in the context of sexual health. The earlier first sex occurs, the less likely it is to be protected. This may reflect a reluctance to seek contraceptive advice or supplies for an act that may be socially prohibited or even against the law. Concerns about confidentiality may also be a deterrent. Issues relating to lack of self-esteem and confidence are important determinants of use. Alternately, failure to protect intercourse can reflect the sporadic nature of sexual activity and somewhat disorganized lives in this age group (see Chapter 3). Some young people find it difficult to accept that they need contraception at all, since they may not intend to have intercourse until it actually occurs. Where there is ambivalence about whether to have sex, the potential for planning and communication is limited and so sexual encounters are more likely to be unprotected.

Contraceptive use varies with context and with age. In western countries, the most common pattern is for condoms to be the first method used, replaced fairly rapidly by the pill. Young people in many contexts may see the risk of pregnancy to be higher than HIV and may lack awareness of other STIs.

Condom use at first sexual intercourse has increased in most countries over recent decades, and in some (such as Uganda) dramatically so. Among single women in 19 African countries, the proportion using a condom at last sex rose from 19% to 28% between 1993 and 2001 (Cleland and Ali, 2006). In general, however, condom use is higher in richer than poorer countries and nowhere is it yet high enough to significantly control the spread of STIs (Wellings et al., 2006).

The social context of young people's sexual behaviour

As noted in Chapter 1, biological factors play a minor role in determining patterns and trends in sexual activity. The correlation between age at first intercourse and age at menarche, for example, is not strong, and the decline in age at menarche has not been on a scale large enough to account for the magnitude of the fall in age at at first intercourse seen in some countries.

In the past, there has been a tendency for research and practice to focus on individual-level influences on young people's behaviour, and on their propensity for risk-taking. This has been termed the 'individual deficit' model, and has been criticized for neglecting the broader social and environmental determinants of risk in young people's lives (Ingham, 2006).

Social change

Trends in young people's sexual behaviour need to be seen against the backcloth of social changes that have taken place in many parts of the world. These include urbanization, high levels of movement and migration, new technologies enabling greater access to information, and disruption to some traditional communities and values. In some contexts, there has been increasing sexualization of society and permissiveness; in others, cultural forces have operated in the opposite direction, and controls on sexual behaviour are tighter.

The second half of the twentieth century also saw marked changes in the education and employment status of women, the advent of effective contraception, and the extension of family planning services in many parts of the world. Demographic trends also help to explain patterns of relationships. Where sexual experience begins earlier, where the time spent in education is longer, and where average age at marriage is rising, young people have longer in which to acquire more sexual partners (Figure 6.2).

Social attitudes

In most societies, social agendas reflect an ambivalence towards the sexuality of young people. This is manifest in attitudes that permit the early sexualization of children via fashion and popular culture, yet at the same time problematize actual sexual behaviour. Discomfort and fear around the sexuality of young people often lead to a focus on negative rather than positive outcomes of sex. The evidence suggests that open and accepting attitudes are associated with positive outcomes such as later sexual debut, less regret about sex, and more consistent contraceptive use (Ingham, 2006). Yet, a pervasive fear is that talking about sex in positive ways with young people will encourage promiscuity. Adopting this view, religious and politically conservative groups have influenced approaches to sex education in several countries (see Chapter 13).

A systematic review of qualitative studies of young people's sexual behaviour found surprising similarities in the nature and direction of social forces shaping young people's behaviour (Marston and King, 2006). Gender stereotypes were crucial in determining social expectations and behaviour and, as we have seen, gendered norms are still extremely strong in many parts of the world.

Internet and media

Much of the media coverage of issues relating to young people is fairly sensationalist. The media routinely inflate levels of sexual activity among young teenagers and thereby create anxiety among the young that they are not keeping up with their peers. Sex on screen rarely portrays concerns with protection, and in many parts of the world depicts women as sex objects and/or as submissive. Such representations can serve to undermine efforts to safeguard young people's sexual health.

Internet access is increasing everywhere and the effects of online influences on young people's sexual health are controversial. Some worry that exposure to pornography leads to desensitization of sexually explicit material and encourages attitudes to sex that are degrading to women; and, more rarely but more seriously, that it exposes young people to sexual predators. Others point to the value of the Internet in providing health-related information, though its value depends on the quality of the website. In fact, what evidence there is suggests that the effects of Internet use may be more modest than is often feared.

Family, friends and religion

Family structure and environment, such as the degree of perceived parental support, exert strong influences on sexual attitudes and behaviour (Vanwesenbeeck et al., 1999). Family disruption has been shown to be associated with earlier intercourse and conception (Wellings et al., 2001). Behaviours and practices witnessed within the family provide influential models, and young people tend to internalize parental attitudes and values (behaving either in accordance or deliberately in opposition). Parents who talk openly with their children about sex can influence behaviour in positive ways, yet many parents find it difficult to do so.

During early adulthood, peers are an important influence on attitudes and behaviour. Much of the interaction occurs within same-sex groups, which generate gender-specific perspectives on issues of sex and relationships. Depending on the friendship group, peer influence may be positive or negative. Social pressure, particularly from peers, is often cited as a reason for young people having intercourse before they feel ready. On the other hand, research also suggests that young men who believe their friends use condoms are more likely to report using them themselves (WHO, 2000).

Many young people grow up in families and communities in which religion shapes identity and determines the dominant value system. Religion can have both a positive and negative impact on young people's sexuality. In strongly religious environments, the benefits of delaying sexual activity may be stressed, but to the neglect of discussion of contraception (Rostosky et al., 2004).

Which young people are most at risk?

Some groups of young people have specific sexual health needs and vulnerabilities, including those in care, those developing alternative sexual identities, HIV positive young people, and those with disabilities. Their heightened risk and vulnerability arise from factors such as lack of self-esteem, experience of stigma and discrimination, lack of protection from significant adults, difficulty accessing services, and lack of knowledge and information.

Activity 6.4

Think about young people infected with HIV perinatally (around the time of birth). What issues do you think they might face? Why do you think they might be vulnerable?

Feedback

It is often during early adulthood that children infected by HIV first come to realize and understand their situation. This realization may spark feelings of anger and resentment (particularly towards their parents), fear and denial. Hopelessness about the future may result in poor adherence to treatment, as there may seem like little point.

Disclosure is a major issue for HIV positive young people: when and how do they tell their friends or a partner about being HIV positive? A culture of silence around appropriate sexual expression for young people living with HIV may result in feelings of fear and confusion. In particular, fear of transmitting HIV to a partner may make it difficult to enjoy sex. HIV positive young people are also vulnerable to stigma and discrimination, not only from their peers but also from adults in authority. There may be concern about confidentiality and a mistrust of healthcare professionals. In countries hardest hit by the AIDS epidemic young people whose parents have died of AIDS may be coming to terms with their status at the same time as heading the household and looking after younger siblings.

Intervention

Interventions for young people aim to: enable young people to begin sexual activity at a time that is ideal for them and in a way that prepares the ground for future safe and satisfying sexual activity; equip them with the skills to resist unwanted sexual advances; and provide them with the means and confidence to protect themselves from unplanned pregnancy and infection.

As we have seen, the sexual behaviour of young people is highly variable. This calls for carefully targeted and tailored interventions to protect their sexual health. The diversity of influences on young people's risk and vulnerability calls for multifaceted approaches. Thus a pregnancy prevention strategy may require involvement from schools, families, social services, and community leaders, as well as health services, to tackle both individual and environmental factors that contribute to unplanned pregnancy. Public health interventions also need to listen to and incorporate the opinions and goals of the young people they purport to serve. The cornerstones of interventions for young people include mass media campaigns, advocacy activities, comprehensive sex education programmes, and youth-friendly sexual health services. These are the focus of Chapters 12, 13, and 14.

Summary

Young people are vulnerable to the adverse consequences of sex as a result of their relative lack of experience, power and autonomy, and access to resources. The variability of behaviour among young people calls for carefully targeted and tailored interventions to protect their sexual health. Social and political agendas relating to young people can undermine attempts to implement evidence-based policy and practice and efforts are needed to mitigate their negative effects.

References

Bearinger LH, Sieving RE, Ferguson J and Sharma V (2007) Global perspectives on the sexual and reproductive health of adolescents: patterns, prevention and potential, *Lancet*, 389: 1220–31.

Biddlecom A, Gregory R, Lloyd CB and Mensch BS (2008) Associations between premarital sex and leaving school in four sub-Saharan African countries, *Studies in Family Planning*, 39(4): 337–50.

Brown A, Jejeebhoy SJ, Shah I and Yount KM (2001) *Sexual Relations Among Young People in Developing Countries: Evidence from WHO Case Studies.* Geneva: WHO. Available at: http://www.who.int/reproductivehealth/publications/adolescence/RHR_01.8/en/index.html

Cleland J and Ali MM (2006) Sexual abstinence, contraception, and condom use by young African women: a secondary analysis of survey data, *Lancet,* 368: 1788–93.

Ingham R (2006) The importance of context in understanding and seeking to promote sexual health, in R. Ingham and P. Aggleton (eds.) *Promoting Young Pople's Sexual Health: International Perspectives.* London: Routledge.

Marston C and King E (2006) Factors that shape young people's sexual behaviour: a systematic review, *Lancet,* 368: 1581–6.

Rostosky S, Wilcox BL, Wright MLC and Randall BA (2004) The impact of religiosity on adolescent sexual behavior: a review of the evidence, *Journal of Adolescent Research,* 19(6): 677–97.

UNICEF (2011) *The State of the World's Children 2011 – Adolescence: An Age of Opportunity.* New York: UNICEF.

Vanwesenbeeck I, van Zessen G, Ingham R, Jaramazovib E and Stevens D (1999) Factors and processes in heterosexual competence and risk: an integrated review of the evidence, *Psychology and Health,* 14(10): 25–50.

Wellings K, Nanchahal K, MacDowall W, McManus S, Erens B, Mercer CH et al. (2001) Sexual behaviour in Britain: early heterosexual experience, *Lancet,* 358: 1843–50.

Wellings K, Collumbien M, Slaymaker E, Singh S, Hodges Z, Patel D et al. (2006) Sexual behaviour in context: a global perspective, *Lancet,* 368: 1706–28.

Wight D and Henderson M (2004) The diversity of young people's heterosexual behaviour, in M Duffy and E Burtney (eds.) *Young People and Sexual Health: Social, Political, and Individual Contexts.* Basingstoke: Palgrave Macmillan.

Wight D, Parkes A, Strange V, Allen E, Bonell C and Henderson M (2008) The quality of young people's heterosexual relationships: a longitudinal analysis of characteristics shaping subjective experience, *Perspectives on Sexual and Reproductive Health,* 40(4): 226–37.

World Health Organization (WHO) (2000) *What about Boys? A Literature Review on the Health and Development of Adolescent Boys.* Geneva: WHO/Pan American Health Organization.

Further reading

Burtney E and Duffy M (eds.) (2004) *Young People and Sexual Health: Individual, Social and Policy Contexts.* Basingstoke: Palgrave Macmillan.

Ingham R and Aggleton P (eds.) (2006) *Promoting Young People's Sexual Health: International Perspectives.* Abingdon: Routledge.

Men who have sex with men

7

Will Nutland and Martine Collumbien

Overview

Men who have sex with men (MSM) are a key target group for sexual health interventions. In this chapter, we first define sexual orientation and sexual identity. We then examine how culture and society shape sexual practice and identity and how same-sex relationships are regulated. We explore why sex between men is treated as a sexual health risk behaviour and why MSM are an important target group for sexual health promotion and services. Finally, we describe challenges relating to providing services and carrying out research with this target group.

Learning outcomes

After reading this chapter, you will be able to:

- Describe how culture and social norms shape identity, behaviour and practice, and how this can change over time
- Explain risk factors and social vulnerabilities affecting MSM in different settings
- Recognize the challenges of implementing public health-orientated research and interventions targeting MSM

Key terms

Hetero-normative: A prevailing assumption that all people feel, identify, and behave as heterosexual.

Sexual identity: How an individual sees and defines their sexual self and how they express that part of themselves to others.

Sexual orientation: The direction of an individual's erotic desire and attraction to partners of the same sex (homosexual), opposite sex (heterosexual), same and opposite sex (bisexual).

Transgender: An individual whose gender identity differs from their sex assigned at birth.

Definitions and categories

Depending on disciplinary perspective, sexual orientation is variously thought to be influenced by biological, psychological, and environmental factors. Of importance from a public health perspective, however, is that sexual orientation is not always fixed and constant, but may be fluid and changing. Instead of fitting neatly into dichotomous categories of exclusively heterosexual and homosexual attraction/experience, individuals tend to occupy positions along a continuum. Survey data from Britain show that 90% of men reporting having had sex with a man also had sex with a woman at some time in their life, and 30% had done so in the last year (NATSAL, unpublished data).

Sexual orientation may vary during the life course. Same-sex attraction might be a singular event in a man's life, for example in sexual experimentation. It might appear later in life; some men marry earlier in life but later 'come out' and adopt an openly gay identity. Same-sex contact may occur fleetingly, according to opportunities available for having male or female partners; in gender-segregated societies, men may engage in homosexual behaviour only before marriage when access to female partners is restricted. It may also be 'situational' where men live in all-male environments such as boarding schools, the army, and prisons.

Not all men who have experienced same-sex sex identify as gay, for a number of reasons. The extent of the 'fit' between sexual expression and sexual identity varies considerably with social context. The concept of a 'gay identity' is not in common currency in many non-western cultures, except among educated urban men with exposure to an international scene or global networks (Asthana and Oostvogels 2001). Even in cultures in which attitudes towards gay men have softened dramatically, not all men with same-sex sexual experience will identify as 'gay'. Some may not associate with the highly commercialized and commodified gay scenes prevalent in western metropoles. Others may have internalized negative messages from their early upbringing and dissociate their sexual practice from an identity they perceive as shameful.

Precisely because people do not always self-identify according to their practices, a focus on behaviours (what people do) is more useful than one on identities (what they see and present themselves as) in a public health context. The term 'men who have sex with men' was introduced in the late twentieth century to describe an epidemiological category of men with behaviours that potentially put them at higher risk of acquiring HIV and other sexually transmitted infections (STIs). The definition accommodates 'a variety of sexual identities as well as those who do not self-identify as homosexual or gay' (UNAIDS, 2006). It remains a contested term, however, with some gay men feeling that being labelled as 'MSM' makes their sexuality invisible or gives an impression that they are marginalized or hard to reach.

Moreover, the category of MSM may be insufficiently discriminating to reflect the nuances of same-sex practice in some settings. In South Asia, for example, labels used to describe categories of men who have sex with men include additional dimensions of sex acts, such as penetrative or receptive, or both. In India, for example, *Kothi* refers to men who prefer the receptive position in sex. These mainly feminized men have developed a strong *Kothi* identity (based on a common stigmatized sexuality); they are a well-networked social group and therefore relatively easy to reach. They label their penetrative partners as *Panthi*, but the majority of these men do not self-identify as such (and hence are harder to reach by interventions). Similar categories are common in Pakistan and Bangladesh and tend to be adopted rigidly by implementers of interventions, belying a more fluid reality regarding sexual roles (Boyce, 2007; Collumbien et al., 2009).

Activity 7.1

Why do you think public health professionals focus on sexual practices rather than sexual identity?

Feedback

Public health professionals are interested in tracking the spread of STIs and assessing the risks of acquiring these diseases both for an individual and within communities. This requires accurate information about activities rather than identities. This is not to say that identity is unimportant in public health. Identity is key to targeting men for intervention. Those who identify as MSM are usually well networked and easy to target, whereas those who do not self-identify are harder to reach.

Attitudes towards homosexuality through time

Same-sex behaviour has existed in most, if not all, societies (Weeks, 1989). Homosexuality is evidenced in ancient texts, religious holy books, art, literature, medical textbooks, and court records. There is documented evidence from the early 1700s, for example, of London's Molly-Houses where men would meet to socialize and have sex, often with 'marriages' taking place between men and their 'girls' (men dressed as women) (Cook, 2007).

Throughout modern history, homosexuality has tended to be defined as deviant and 'unnatural' and as being in particular need of regulation. In England, the earliest law regulating sexual behaviour between men was the law against all non-procreative sexual 'acts'. These acts, notably that of sodomy, were punishable by death, and later by life imprisonment. This was replaced by two years' hard labour, introduced in the 1885 Criminal Law Amendment Act, a more lenient penalty but one that was more commonly enforced. Famous trials, such as the trial of playwright Oscar Wilde, served to demonstrate publicly that the law regarded homosexual acts as deviant behaviour. Paradoxically, such prosecutions led other men with homosexual leanings to become more self-conscious about their orientation, to self-define as homosexual, and to adopt an outward identity (Weeks, 1989). Control of same-sex relationships has focused on men rather than women. There are few instances in any society of lesbian sex being the focus of legislation.

The late nineteenth century saw increasing engagement of the medical establishment in the regulation of homosexuality. Contemporary scientific discussions focused on whether or not it could be cured. Treatments ranged from hypnosis to aversion therapy, in some cases involving electric shock therapy (Cook, 2007). These treatments were at best ineffective and at worst harmful. Not until 1973 did the American Psychiatric Association remove homosexuality from the Diagnostic and Statistical Manual of Mental Disorders (DSM), following an impassioned debate. Psychiatrists were compelled to confront the issue as a result of political activism by the gay liberation movement – an example of how pressure from civil society can bring about change.

In the final decades of the twentieth century, HIV had a huge impact on attitudes towards homosexuality. In the early days of the AIDS epidemic, panic about HIV led to a backlash against gay communities. In many western countries, this ultimately led to a greater resilience and a stronger reshaping of a gay identity, accompanied by greater social tolerance and integration, rather than further repression of homosexual behaviour. Activism by civil rights groups influenced the policy debate and community-based organizations were formed to provide health education, promote safer sex and, importantly, to campaign for political responses to HIV/AIDS.

Attitudes towards homosexuality across cultures

In most Western societies, radical changes in social attitudes to same-sex activity have led to legal protection and improved rights. Many parts of the world now have anti-discrimination laws providing protection in the workplace and in the provision of goods and services for gay men and lesbians; an equal age of consent for heterosexual and homosexual sex; and legislation to enact same-sex marriage or civil partnerships. These changes have not been confined to North America and Europe. In South Africa, equality for lesbians and gay men is enshrined within the constitution, and same-sex marriage has been legalized in Brazil and Argentina in recent years.

Yet homosexuality remains criminalized in over 80 countries of the world. Half of these are Commonwealth countries where homosexuality was prohibited under sodomy law introduced during British rule. In India, homosexual activity was considered acceptable before colonization. In China, it was regarded as a normal facet of life prior to the spread of Christian and Islamic values via Central Asia. Homosexuality was then banned in the People's Republic of China, until it was legalized in 1997. The definition given for sodomy in the Indian penal code of 1860 was: 'Whoever voluntarily has carnal intercourse against the order of nature with any man, woman or animal ...'. Language such as 'order of nature' reflects the essentialist assumption that certain acts are natural and others are not (see Chapter 1).

At the time of writing, there has been something of an escalation of anti-homosexual sentiment in some African countries. In Uganda, draft legislation for an Anti-Homosexuality Bill proposed the death penalty for same-sex activity in 2009. In Malawi, a sentence of 14 years in prison with hard labour was imposed in 2010 on a gay couple convicted of gross indecency after holding an engagement ceremony. Whether or not enacted, such legislation creates a climate of fear and intimidation that makes it difficult for men to express their sexuality openly. Instead, many are forced to live a double life and hide their sexuality from their family. They may marry women and continue to have sex with men in secret (Cáceres et al., 2009). Under these conditions, prevalent in most of Africa and in Muslim countries in the Middle East, the implementation of sexual health programmes among MSM is severely compromised.

In Latin America and parts of Asia, laws are less prohibitive but social regulation still leads to stigmatization and human rights violations. Research and sexual health interventions are possible only among the most visible groups of MSM, usually effeminate men and transgender persons. At the same time, the very fact of their visibility exposes these groups to further discrimination with little recourse to protection from the State (Cáceres et al., 2009).

Within and across religions, positions on homosexuality vary widely. While some faith communities embrace homosexuals within their congregations and support gay and lesbian faith leaders, others remain vehemently opposed to same-sex behaviour. For example, in some parts of the USA, openly gay men have been ordained as Anglican Bishops; in other parts, churches campaign globally to protect traditional heterosexual family values and the sanctity of marriage, campaigns that resonate among some African congregations.

Activity 7.2

History suggests that attitudes towards homosexuality within a culture can and do shift over time. Think about your own culture. What factors influence public opinion? Can you think of any specific events that have brought about a shift in attitudes in the recent past?

Feedback

Attitudes may shift following a key event such as a celebrity 'coming out' or a scandal or series of arrests or prosecutions, murders or hate crimes. Shifts may be driven or supported by the media (newspapers, television, Internet). Religious leaders may call for a greater understanding of homosexuality or, conversely, for a moral 'crack down' on same-sex sex. Activism by civil rights groups may influence the policy debate and bring about changes in legislation. Changes to the law, in turn, may influence social attitudes either negatively or positively. Internet and other media technologies facilitate communication between and about gay people, gay sex, and gay lifestyles. The globalization of 'western gay culture' and increased networking can support MSM to advocate for change in their own countries.

MSM and sexual health

Across Western Europe, North America, and Australia, MSM make up a large proportion of people living with HIV (Sahasrabuddhe and Vermund, 2009). In the UK and USA, over half of new HIV infections are homosexually acquired (Centers for Disease Control, 2010; Health Protection Agency, 2010), and outbreaks of syphillis and *Lymphogranuloma venereum* (LGV) in Europe in the last decade were predominantly in groups of gay men (Van de Laar, 2006).

In low- and middle-income countries, MSM have a greater risk of acquiring HIV compared with men who do not have sex with men. Even in Africa, the incidence of HIV is higher among MSM. In Kenya and Zambia, the prevalence among MSM is 15% and 33% respectively; both rates are double that of the general population (Godwin, 2010). In Ghana where HIV in the general population is relatively low at 1.7% of the general population, it is 25% among MSM (Godwin, 2010).

Men who have sex with men can also be at higher risk of experiencing sexual violence because of their sexual identity. The risk is higher in contexts in which sex between men is highly stigmatized and/or illegal, and in which violence against MSM is condoned. Intimate partner violence has also been reported in same-sex relationships, with the victim usually the man taking the receptive role in sex (see Chapter 4).

Sexual ill health impacts differentially across different groups of MSM. In the UK, men with lower levels of education, younger men, and Black men all have greater HIV prevention needs (CHAPS Partnership, 2011). Globally, MSM who are migrants, asylum seekers or refugees are likely to have enhanced vulnerability to sexual ill health (see Chapter 9).

Activity 7.3

What might be the reasons for the greater incidence of HIV and STIs among MSM?

Feedback

- In contexts in which sex between men is illegal or MSM are marginalized, men might be reluctant to access STI treatment services for fear of discrimination. In addition, MSM often carry a greater burden of mental health and behavioural problems – such as depression, drug and alcohol misuse, and violence – which can impact on the control they have over their sex lives, health, and well-being (Stall et al., 2009).
- MSM tend to have higher rates of partner exchange, thereby increasing the likelihood of HIV and STI acquisition and transmission. And since HIV and STI prevalence is already greater amongst MSM, sex between men will carry a greater risk.
- Anal intercourse carries a greater risk of HIV and STI transmission than vaginal or oral intercourse because of physiological vulnerability. The membranes of the anus and rectum are more delicate and less well lubricated, compared with the vagina, and resultant abrasions allow a direct entry to the body by infective organisms.
- 'Role versatility', whereby men adopt both 'insertive' and 'receptive' roles, may also play a part, since infection can occur through unprotected receptive sex, and infect a subsequent partner through insertive sex.

Before the advent of anti-retroviral therapies, strategies such as condom use and negotiated safety (whereby HIV negative partners in a regular partnership agree to dispense with condoms within the relationship but to adhere to safe sex with other partners) had some success in lowering HIV incidence among gay men in western countries. The wider availability of highly active anti-retroviral therapy (HAART) resulted initially in a decline in HIV diagnoses among gay men, followed by an increase in HIV notification rates, which could not be explained by changes in HIV testing alone (Sullivan et al., 2009). This reversal provides a good illustration of the challenges of maintaining consistent safer sex behaviour across a population (de Wit et al., 2011). It showed that, to be effective, public health interventions need to maintain the focus on prevention.

Research among MSM

Accurate information on the risk and risk reduction behaviour among MSM is essential to public health intervention and to advocacy. For example, as we saw above, lesbianism attracts less moral outrage, perhaps because what women do sexually together is seen as less morally offensive, since it does not include penile-anal intercourse (Weeks, 1989). The equation of 'homosexual' with 'anal' sex among men is common among lay and health professionals alike. Yet an Internet survey of over 180,000 MSM across Europe (EMIS, 2011) showed that oral sex was most commonly practised, followed by mutual masturbation, with anal intercourse in third place.

The social climate in a country, however, determines the extent to which reliable estimates of same-sex behaviour can be obtained. Individuals may be reluctant to report behaviour they think is perceived to be deviant or stigmatized. They may not acknowledge their behaviour to themselves, let alone report it in a survey. Surveillance is likely to underestimate homosexually acquired sexual infections if sexual activity between men is illegal or socially stigmatized (Baral et al., 2007).

In countries in which homosexuality is criminalized, questions about same-sex activity are rarely asked in general population samples. A systematic review of HIV risk in low- and middle-income countries found that apart from Mexico, Brazil, Thailand, and Peru, lower-income countries had not systematically surveyed their populations of MSM (Baral et al., 2007). International funding bodies for HIV prevention have encouraged research amongst MSM using special sampling methods to reach hidden groups (see Chapter 15). This research remains sensitive and requires careful risk assessment to protect researchers and participants alike.

Activity 7.4

Consider why men taking part in a survey might not answer a question about same-sex experience.

Feedback

Reasons might include:

- a mistrust of the researcher or agency undertaking the survey, together with fears about confidentiality of data;
- the ways in which respondents view their sexual identity and practices; for example, some may not acknowledge their same-sex activity as 'sex';
- differences in what 'counts' as a sexual encounter make it difficult to measure the extent of same-sex practice and experience;
- sexual encounters that occurred some time ago may be discounted as 'insignificant', as might those that did not involve penetration.

Sexual health interventions for MSM

Public health interventions are needed that address structural determinants of risk and vulnerabilities for MSM. The aim should be one of creating an enabling environment – one in which men are able to achieve sexual health status according to the WHO definition (see Chapter 1). This includes removal of legal barriers that undermine access to HIV-related services, promoting and guaranteeing human rights, and training and sensitizing healthcare providers to avoid discriminating against MSM.

Effective interventions will comprise a number of key components. Health promotion materials need to have targeted information on prevention and risk reduction strategies, designed to appeal to and meet the needs of MSM. Safe spaces or drop-in centres are needed to enable MSM to access services. Health services that are 'MSM-friendly', with well-trained staff who respect confidentiality, are more likely to be accessed by MSM. At a minimum, such services should provide condoms and water-based lubricants, confidential, voluntary HIV screening and care, and management of STIs. As an ideal they would also include counselling services to address sexual function problems, experiences of sexual violence, and feelings around sexual identity.

As we have seen, MSM are not a homogenous group and it is important that interventions do not frame them as such. Health promotion activities need to be tailored to culturally specific needs of MSM. Within the same country, sexually explicit imagery might work well for some groups (urban, confident clubbers) but may be unacceptable to others (such as married men). Promotional material suited to a gay bar or pub may be less so in other contexts, such as sexual health clinics.

There is evidence that the use of the media in public health campaigns can serve to increase tolerance in relation to MSM. One example is a popular Lebanese TV series that included gay voices when discussing sexuality, even though their faces were hidden behind masks (Hélie, 2004). Another example is a popular Pakistani transgender chat show host who gained a fan club of Pakistani politicians, film stars, and army dignitaries who appear as guests on the show (*The Independent*, 2009).

Pleas have been made to avoid a narrow focus on STI acquisition (including HIV). The gay men's health movement has called for such 'deficit models' of MSM health to be challenged, arguing that shame and guilt about (homo)sex and (homo)sexuality are the real health hazards. Some have argued that the ability to experiment, love, and explore sexuality in a multitude of ways is healthy, affirming, and celebratory (Rofes, 1996). For public health practitioners, attempts to reduce the harm of HIV, STIs, and sexual ill health in MSM, alongside efforts to protect sexual fulfilment and enjoyment among MSM can be a fine balance, not least if government funding and policy require evidence of reductions in disease incidence.

One example of the adoption of a broader sexual health framework, which promotes sex as a positive and enriching force, was developed in the UK by a partnership of well-established organizations seeking to improve the sexual health of MSM with funding from the Department of Health. A key principle of the framework is that 'all men have the right to express and enjoy their sexuality'. The framework is rooted in the concept of benefits-driven change – a belief that it is possible for MSM to experience both an improvement in their sex lives and a reduction in the harm arising from their sex lives (CHAPS Partnership, 2011).

Summary

Attitudes towards same-sex behaviour, as well as their specific social meanings, vary widely across time and across cultures, and need to be considered in their historical context. Men who have sex with men are a key target group for sexual health interventions. They are not a homogeneous group and some sub-populations of MSM will have greater sexual health needs than others. In many societies, same-sex relationships are criminalized and this strongly influences the approaches that public health interventions and research can take. Interventions to improve the sexual health of MSM need to take into account the benefits as well as the costs of sex and need to be tailored according to setting and cultural and legal context. Researching sexual behaviour among MSM is challenging, not least because some men are reluctant to report same-sex activity or are unwilling to view that activity as being 'sex'.

References

Asthana S and Oostvogels R (2001) The social construction of male homosexuality in India: implications for HIV transmission and prevention, *Social Science and Medicine*, 52: 707–21.

Baral S, Sifakis F, Cleghorn F and Beyrer C (2007) Elevated risk for HIV infection among men who have sex with men in low and middle income countries 2000–2006: a systematic review, *PLoS Medicine*, 4(12): e339.

Boyce P (2007) 'Conceiving Khotis': men who have sex with men in India and the cultural subject of HIV prevention, *Medical Anthropology*, 26: 175–203.

Cáceres CF, Pecheny M, Frasca T, Rios RR and Pocahy F (2009) *Review of Legal Frameworks and the Situation of Human Rights Related to Sexual Diversity in Low and Middle Income Countries*. Geneva: UNAIDS.

Centers for Disease Control (2010) *HIV among Gay, Bisexual and Other Men who have Sex with Men (MSM)*, September 2010. Atlanta, GA: Centers for Disease Control. Available at: http://www.cdc.gov/hiv/topics/msm/pdf/msm.pdf.

CHAPS Partnership (2011) *Making it Count 4: A Collaborative Planning Framework to Minimise the Incidence of HIV Infection during Sex between Men*, 4th edn. London: Sigma Research.

Collumbien M, Qureshi AA, Mayhew SH, Rizvi N, Rabbani A, Rolfe B et al. (2009) Understanding the context of male and transgender sex work using peer ethnography, *Sexually Transmitted Infections*, 85(suppl.): ii3–ii7.

Cook M (2007) *A Gay History of Britain – Love and Sex between Men since the Middle Ages*. Oxford: Greenwood.

de Wit JBF, Aggleton P, Myers T and Crewe M (2011) The rapidly changing paradigm of HIV prevention: time to strengthen social and behavioural approaches, *Health Education Research*, 26(3): 381–92.

EMIS (2011) *The European MSM Internet Survey (EMIS) – Community Report 2*. Available at: http://www.emis-project.eu/sites/default/files/public/publications/emis-community2_english_4.pdf.

Godwin J (2010) *Enabling Legal Environments for Effective HIV Responses: A Leadership Challenge for the Commonwealth*. Available at: http://www.aidsalliance.org/publicationsdetails.aspx?id=496.

Health Protection Agency (2010) *HIV in the United Kingdom: 2010 Report*. London: Health Protection Agency. Available at: http://www.hpa.org.uk/web/HPAwebFile/HPAweb_C/1287145367237.

Hélie A (2004) Holy hatred, *Reproductive Health Matters*, 12(23): 120–4.

Rofes E (1996) *Reviving the Tribe: Regenerating Gay Men's Sexuality and Culture in the Ongoing Epidemic*. Binghamton, NY: Harrington Park Press.

Sahasrabuddhe VV and Vermund SH (2009) Current and future trends: implications for HIV prevention, in KH Mayer and HF Pizer (eds.) *HIV Prevention – A Comprehensive Approach*. London: Academic Press.

Stall R, Herrick A, Guadamuz T and Friedman M (2009) Updating HIV prevention with gay men: current challenges and opportunities to advance health among gay men, in KH Mayer and HF Pizer (eds.) *HIV Prevention – A Comprehensive Approach*. London: Academic Press.

Sullivan PS, Hamouda O, Delpech V, Geduld JE, Prejean J, Semaille C et al. (2009) Reemergence of the HIV epidemic among men who have sex with men in North America, Western Europe, and Australia, 1996–2005, *Annals of Epidemiology*, 19: 423–31.

The Independent (2009) http://www.independent.co.uk/news/world/asia/lifes-a-drag-act-for-the-tv-presenter-challenging-homophobia-in-pakistan-1825925.html.

UNAIDS (2006) *UNAIDS Policy Brief: HIV and Sex between Men*, August 2006. Geneva: UNAIDS. Available at: http://www.unaids.org/en/media/unaids/contentassets/dataimport/pub/briefingnote/2006/20060801_policy_brief_msm_en.pdf.

Van de Laar MJ (2006) The emergence of LGV in Western Europe: what do we know, what can we do?, *Eurosurveillance*, 11(9): pii=641. Available at: http://www.eurosurveillance.org/ViewArticle. aspx?ArticleId=641.

Weeks J (1989) *Sex, Politics and Society*, 2nd edn. London: Longmans.

Further reading

Global Forum on MSM and HIV (2010) *HIV Prevention with MSM – Balancing Evidence with Rights-based Principles of Practice: A Policy Brief*, June 2010. Oakland, CA: MSMGF. Available at: www.msmgf.org.

Weeks J (1989) The construction of homosexuality, in *Sex, Politics and Society*, 2nd edn. London: Longmans.

Sex workers 8

Elisabeth Pisani

Overview

Sex work is associated with significant occupational risks, particularly with regard to sexual health. In this chapter, we discuss reasons for buying and selling sex, and describe some of the diversity in the industry. We examine the perspectives and assumptions that underlie the way societies deal with sex work, discuss the occupational and sexual health needs of sex workers, and describe some of the intervention approaches that can meet these needs.

Learning outcomes

After reading this chapter, you will be able to:

- Describe the diversity of people who sell sex and the social contexts in which sex work takes place
- Critically examine assumptions underlying societal responses to sex work
- Recognize the occupational health issues facing sex workers, particularly with regard to sexual health
- Describe the major interventions that promote health among commercial sex workers

Key terms

Abolitionism: A movement that seeks to eradicate prostitution.

Occupational health: Health issues and needs that arise specifically from a person's working environment and practices.

Sex worker: In this chapter, a sex worker is defined as a person who sells sex for cash or drugs, with no further expectation or commitment between buyer and seller.

Defining sex work

The first challenge in discussing sex workers is to define them. The very language we use is laden with values, which can determine how we, as a society, view sex work, and thus how we approach it. The term 'prostitution' is used in law enforcement and when arguing for and against criminalization of sex work. It is a term generally used by people who believe that the sale of sex for money can never be a legitimate form of work.

Although regarded as insulting by some, a number of sex worker organizations in the West have recently re-appropriated the term. In global public health, the term 'sex work' is most current. In this chapter, the terms 'sex worker' and 'prostitution' are both used, attaching no moral or political judgement to them.

Whatever term is used, it is often not clear to whom it refers. There is general agreement that people who accept cash in exchange for a single, pre-agreed act of sex are sex workers, and in early surveys of sexual behaviour, any sex in exchange for 'money, gifts or favours' was classified as commercial. But what about people who take payment in other forms, such as drugs or rent? How should we classify strippers and porn stars who do not sell sex but call themselves sex workers?

Activity 8.1

Write down all the reasons why people have sex. How many of these involve an actual or implicit exchange of money, gifts or favours? What criteria can you use to decide if sex that involves exchange is actually sex work?

Feedback

Your list might include some of the following: pleasure; it is their job; their partner just paid for a nice dinner; their spouse wants to; they hope their partner will pay their rent or school-fees; they get raped; they want a baby; they want free drugs; they want to relieve stress; they want to express their love to their partner; and so on.

Reasons such as a request for rent, school-fees or drugs, or payback for dinner include an explicit or implicit exchange. However, it is usually only people who take cash in exchange for sex who are thought of as sex workers. In this chapter, sex workers are defined as people who sell sex for cash or drugs, with no further expectation or commitment between buyer and seller.

Who's who in sex work – the oldest profession?

Sex work has existed throughout history, and in most cultures. Attitudes towards the exchange of sex for money vary with different societies and cultures, through time, and for men and women.

In most pre-industrial societies, men had to accumulate resources before they could acquire a wife, preferably one at the start of her childbearing years. This obligation gave rise to social norms and customs including: large age differences at marriage; an expectation of female virginity at marriage; and strong lifelong controls over women's sexuality. Most societies were more tolerant of men's need for sexual fulfilment. This created an imbalance: men not yet rich enough to marry were expected to have sex, whereas unmarried women were not. This gap was often filled by prostitutes. Prostitutes also filled a need when there was a lack of physical attraction within a marriage, which was often the case where arranged marriages were the norm.

This pattern persists in many societies today particularly where, historically, women's freedom of movement has been limited, as in many countries in Asia and Latin America.

In these societies, female sex work is often highly organized, with a high proportion of women working in brothels, massage parlours, and bars known to have sex on sale, even where sex work is technically illegal. In some countries, persistent campaigns warning against unprotected sex with sex workers may have provided the impetus to greater acceptance of premarital sex (Monitoring the AIDS Pandemic, 2004).

In societies in which women have traditionally enjoyed greater freedom of movement (for example, interacting with men in education or at work), the sex trade tends to be less organized and less formal. In many countries in Africa and Europe, for example, there are fewer brothels, and a higher proportion of women sell sex on a freelance basis, often only occasionally. The boundary between commercial and casual partners can be harder to define.

Male and transgender sex workers are more likely than female sex workers to work on a freelance basis and their social role varies. In countries where homosexuality is rarely openly expressed and/or where the pressure to marry and have children is strong, men who are sexually attracted to other men may find it convenient to pay for sex with a male sex worker. The clients of transgender sex workers are more likely to be heterosexual men in search of variety; or men who want anal sex but dare not ask a woman for it; or, where male sex workers are much cheaper (as in Pakistan), men who cannot afford a female sex worker.

Who sells sex?

Globally, the majority of the people who sell sex are women, though in some cities, such as London, it is estimated that up to 40% are men (Scambler and Paoli, 2008). The majority of male sex workers sell sex to other men, some only sell sex to women, and some do both. A male sex worker's clients do not necessarily reflect his own sexual preferences. Many men who sell sex to other men have non-paying partners who are women.

A high proportion of transgendered men – those born as a man but living life as a woman – sell sex in many societies, though the absolute number is small.

A commonly held assumption is that people sell sex because they have to – either they have been tricked or forced into the job against their will. This is certainly true for some sex workers, but the proportion appears to be small in every case where there has been a systematic attempt to evaluate it. In 2009, for example, police in the UK raided over 800 brothels but were unable to find more than a handful of sex workers who had been coerced into their work (Davies, 2009). In some cases in Asia, women 'rescued' from brothels have escaped from centres in which they were being taught other skills and have chosen to go back to sex work (Pisani, 2008).

Many sex workers report being forced to sell sex because no other work is available. Some exaggerate their destitution because poverty is seen as an 'acceptable' motivation for an otherwise unacceptable career choice (Pickering et al., 1992). Certainly, it may be hard for women with limited qualifications to find other jobs that pay as well as sex work. In Vietnam, Cambodia, and Nepal, sex workers report earning up to seven times more than the general population in the same area. Calculating earnings per hours worked, the gap is substantial. In Indonesia, factory workers earned less than 20 US cents an hour on average at a time when even street and brothel-based sex workers (the lowest earners) were averaging US$8 an hour (Pisani, 2008: 217).

Sex workers meet clients in different ways. High-end sex workers use agencies to introduce them to often high-ranking individuals who pay large sums of money in exchange for sex. Many sex workers, especially men, meet clients on the Internet; this is common in developing countries with a limited gay scene. Female sex workers increasingly favour networks that use mobile phones as a point of contact. All these points of contact are more efficient and safer than the street, and are associated with higher earnings.

Despite the diversity in types of sex work, the image of the street-walker continues to dominate popular perceptions of sex work. Another common belief is that most sex workers are drug addicts. In fact, street-based sex workers are more likely to be selling sex to fund a drug habit than are those working in other settings. In cities in the former Soviet Union, for example, between 25 and 80 percent of female sex workers are estimated to be regular drug injectors, with the highest levels among those on the streets (Lowndes et al., 2003). In many cities, sex workers who appear to be drug users are often barred from indoor and cooperative sex work organizations (Plumridge and Abel, 2001). They end up on the street where the sex market and drug market is often so strongly intertwined that continued drug use seems inescapable (Inciardi and Surratt, 2001). In resource-poor countries, patterns of drug consumption among sex workers vary widely. In many countries (including China and some Latin American and Central Asian countries), high proportions of female drug injectors sell sex. However, again, the overall numbers are small. In China, for example, national surveillance data show that some 40% of female injectors report selling sex, yet under 10% of all female sex workers report injecting drugs.

Activity 8.2

Write down what you think might be the reasons why someone would sell sex, and why someone would buy it. Do the reasons differ according to gender? Can you think of any ways in which self-reported motivations may be biased?

Feedback

The most commonly cited reasons for selling sex (as indeed for doing most jobs) are economic. Transgendered men and women, and women are more likely to report that they have no other way of earning a living. Men are more likely to say selling sex is a relatively easy way to earn money.

Limited research has explored why men buy sex, and virtually none why women do so. Paid sex is convenient in that it satisfies a desire for sex without the need for seduction, and need not involve an ongoing relationship. However, some clients do primarily seek friendship and intimacy (known as GFE – the girlfriend experience), and relationships between sex workers and their clients can be close as well as long term (Sanders, 2008). Sex work allows people to explore fantasies and sex acts they may be embarrassed to share with a regular partner. It relieves loneliness and boredom, especially for those working away from home (Hammond, 2010). It provides physical contact for those who might find it hard to obtain it (such as the disabled). And it provides access to partners of genders, races or physique that might otherwise be hard to secure. More than one of these reasons may be relevant to each individual client.

Almost all data on motivations for selling or buying sex are based on self-report, and so do not always accurately reflect 'reality'. Reported motivations may be affected by desire to present oneself in a positive light or by the need to protect oneself. In many European countries, for example, foreigners arrested for selling sex willingly can be deported. However, if they report that they are victims of trafficking, they may be granted asylum or state help. This may lead to an over-reporting of coercion.

Societal perspectives on sex work

Society's views on prostitution heavily influence the approaches public health workers can take to providing sexual health and other services for sex workers. There are two main ways of thinking about sex work, both of which profoundly impact on the lives of sex workers and their clients. The first, sometimes known as abolitionism, holds that sex work is inherently violent and degrading, and must be wiped out. The second centres on harm reduction: in this case, sex work is seen as inevitable, and should be made as safe as any other job.

Prostitution equals violence

Some believe that anyone who buys sex is committing an act of violence against the person selling sex. According to this view, since the sale of sex is inherently degrading, it is impossible for anyone to do it willingly. This perspective underlies the Swedish government's position on sex work: 'No prostitution can be said to be voluntary', stated the Swedish *Study on Prostitution*, which preceded the 1999 Law on the Purchase of Sex. Swedish law makes buying sex a criminal offence. By arresting buyers of sex rather than sellers, the law hopes to eliminate demand for paid sex. Many countries are following the Swedish example. The approach finds favour with conservative religious leaders who see prostitution as a moral issue, as well as with politically liberal feminists. These unlikely allies hope to abolish prostitution in the same way that slavery was abolished in much of the world in the nineteenth century.

Sex work as just another job

Sex workers' rights groups reject the comparison between the abolition of slavery and that of sex work, holding that while no-one chose to be a slave, many people choose to sell sex. Many believe that there is nothing inherently exploitative about sex work provided both seller and buyer agree willingly to the transaction. It is not the exchange of sex for money that is the cause of risks and problems, but 'the poor conditions under which that exchange takes place' (Chapkis, 2011:330). Sex work has continued to exist in some form in most human societies, despite many attempts to prohibit it. Those who believe that there will always be both a demand for, and willing supply of, sex for money argue that abolitionist laws make things worse by driving the whole industry underground and making it harder to identify cases of true coercion.

People who view sex work as a legitimate employment choice believe societies should do all they can to make it safe. This means removing criminal penalties for both buyers and sellers, and providing structures and services that will reduce violence and the risk of infection. New Zealand and Germany are prominent examples of countries that have taken a harm reduction approach to sex work.

The health needs of sex workers

Public health concerns relating to the sex industry largely, although not exclusively, focus on sexually transmitted infections (STIs), including HIV. Both sex workers and their clients may need specific services to reduce the potential for exposure to STIs as well as to treat infections that do occur, since their larger number of partners puts them at increased risk.

Sex workers' sexual health needs fall into two categories. First, occupational health services are needed to help people do their jobs well and safely. Second, sex workers have sexual and reproductive health needs associated with their lives as private citizens.

It is important to recognize that the health risks posed by sex work are highly context-dependent. Data from national surveillance systems suggests that in many industrial countries only street-based sex workers are at higher risk of HIV; the great majority of sex workers who work indoors in the UK, Germany, and Canada, for example, are no more likely to be infected with HIV than school teachers of the same age and gender. In other countries, for example Indonesia, infection rates among sex workers exceed those among other people in the population 100-fold (Ministry of Health, 2009). Within a given country, female, male, and transgender sex workers will face different risks, and will have different needs. The types of risk and the services required will differ dramatically according to the legal and cultural climate of their country, the place of sex work, the type of client, and other factors. The specific conditions of the sex market (whether street-based and run by pimps/drug dealers or premises controlled by gatekeeper colleagues) are particularly important in determining the risk of harm (Cusick, 2006).

Occupational health and safety

Since sex workers need willing buyers, one of their primary concerns is maintaining a level of sexual health that will not deter clients. The prevention of both pregnancy and STIs, and the prompt treatment of the latter, are priorities for sex workers. Infections that are symptomatic (such as bacterial vaginosis) may impact more on earnings than those that are less so (such as HIV) and so may be of more immediate concern to sex workers. Asymptomatic STIs in women may be symptomatic in male clients, who are then unlikely to return.

High-quality STI screening services are important. Since STIs can be transmitted via anal and oral sex, and since these STIs are often asymptomatic, sex workers need services that screen for STIs in the rectum and the throat as well as the vagina and/or urethra. This is especially true for male and transgender sex workers. There are many different approaches to STI screening and treatment (see Chapter 2). Choosing the appropriate strategy for sex workers will depend on the background prevalence of STIs, client turnover, levels of condom use, and the resources available for diagnostic tests, physical examinations, and medications.

The most effective form of STI and HIV prevention for people who sell sex and their clients is the consistent use of condoms. While it is often said that clients will pay more for unprotected sex, large data sets collected from both sex workers and clients show no difference in the amount paid in the last transaction according to whether a condom was used or not.[1] In countries where condom use in commercial sex is relatively low, the strongest determinant of whether or not a female sex worker used a condom with her last client is whether she asked her client to use a condom (Pisani, 2008: 211). But whether or not a sex worker has the agency to make such a request will depend on her perceived power relative to her client, in turn a factor of her working conditions.

Condom use is typically higher in commercial sex than in any other type of sexual encounter; this is true for all genders and for anal as well as vaginal sex. In an analysis of large-scale surveillance in many countries, over 80% of both sex workers and their clients said they use condoms in every transaction.[2] Where condom use in commercial sex is low, it is often at least in part because the most basic interventions have not been put in place; condoms are not freely available at the time and place where sex happens. High levels of alcohol use (by both sex worker and client) are also often correlated with low condom use.

The use of water-based lubricant can also reduce the risk of rectal or vaginal trauma, thus reducing the risk for HIV and other STI transmission. Interventions targeting male and transgender sex workers typically include the provision of lubricant; those targeting female sex workers rarely do, even though natural vaginal lubrication is the result of a sexual arousal that sex workers rarely feel for their clients.

Activity 8.3

Selling sex for a living carries risks for other aspects of health. What do you think these might be?

Feedback

As mentioned, many sex workers have addictions that may require attention and treatment. Some are exposed to harassment and violence (see Chapter 4), especially where sex work is criminalized, and robbery and rape are not uncommon. In some countries, it is common for police to demand free sex in exchange for not arresting a sex worker. Mental health is also a concern, though one that is rarely met.

Personal sexual health needs

Most sex workers make a clear distinction between their professional and their personal lives. One of the ways in which they do so is by using condoms with clients but not with husbands, boyfriends or lovers. This can be difficult, as some regular clients transition into 'boyfriends' without actually reducing their own risk of exposure to STIs or HIV from other sources.

Most female sex workers try to avoid pregnancy while working. Effective contraception that does not involve or affect clients in any way is important, though it is often not provided by sex worker-specific services. Services for sex workers can be unwelcoming, leaving an important gap in providing for sex workers' needs (see Chapter 14). If clinic staff are judgemental, many sex workers prefer to self-diagnose and self-medicate. This has contributed to antibiotic-resistant strains of STIs in many countries.

Intervention approaches

There are two main approaches to promoting sexual health among sex workers. The first is to work with individual sex workers, to support healthy behaviours (individual approach); the second is to alter the context in which sex work takes place (structural approach). Structural interventions include 'bottom-up' empowerment approaches that use collective action by groups of sex workers to change the distribution of power. They also include 'top-down' macro-level interventions that seek to effect legal and structural changes at the level of the sex industry as a whole (see Chapter 12).

Individual approaches often take the form of 'peer outreach'. Following training in sexual health outreach, sex workers are tasked with discussing condom use with colleagues and referring them to STI screening and treatment services. They seek not only to improve knowledge but also to increase negotiating skills. The approach is based on the premise that 'insider' outreach workers have a better understanding of the realities and limitations of the sex worker environment than 'outsider' health professionals. The success of outreach-based programmes has been mixed. They have been mostly successful at increasing condom use in more affluent contexts where sex workers are already linked through networks based on common identity and solidarity. They tend to fail when sex workers see each other as business rivals, where sex workers are marginalized and lack agency, where there is high mobility, and when important others are not supportive. An example of the latter is bar owners encouraging alcohol use by both client and sex worker, thus inhibiting condom negotiation (Campbell and Cornish, 2010).

Empowerment approaches, such as community mobilization, have evolved from peer-based approaches but they view the locus of change as situated within the community context rather than with the individual. In particular, they seek to change relationships of power within the social context (Evans et al., 2009). The Sonagachi project among sex workers in Calcutta is a prominent example. Central to Sonagachi's success was the fact that sex workers were not treated as beneficiaries. Instead, intervention strategies emphasized sex workers' representation, active participation, and empowerment to act collectively. The aim was to reduce vulnerability, increase collective agency, and create healthy peer norms (Jana et al., 2004; Evans et al., 2009). These approaches use critical thinking, community dialogue, and debate. They also involve sex workers in the community in negotiations with police, brothel owners, and health providers to create health-enhancing environments (Campbell and Cornish, 2010). The social and political context in Calcutta was particularly favourable; trade unions are widespread and the local community is familiar with the idea of protest movements and solidarity. Facilitating successful alliances with outside groups who have the power to advance sex workers' interests is thought to be crucial. Without simultaneous support from these important constituencies, empowerment approaches are unlikely to succeed (Campbell and Cornish, 2010).

One of the most famous examples of a 'structural' approach at the macro-level is the '100 percent condom' campaign that originated in Northern Thailand in 1991. Sex work is illegal in Thailand. It is also very common. The Thai Government was alarmed by high rates of HIV among sex workers and evidence that close to a quarter of Thai men bought sex. They asked brothel owners to ensure that clients used condoms and checked up on this by screening all sex workers for STIs fortnightly. They also asked all men presenting with STIs which brothels they had been using. Infections provided evidence that the brothel owner was not enforcing condom use; the offending brothel was then shut down. This implied an end to the livelihoods of both the brothel owner and the sex workers. Though some sex workers' rights groups later complained that the policy was coercive, it was effective. Condom use in commercial sex venues rose dramatically and both STIs and new HIV infections plunged (Celentano et al., 1998). The implementation of this government policy required high-level coordination between different ministries, the media, and law enforcement. It also relied on existing sophisticated STI clinic systems. Although it was difficult to replicate the Thailand programme in its entirety, a study in the Dominican Republic compared interventions in two regions. The intervention was significantly more effective where empowerment approaches were supplemented with government policies on condom use that put responsibility on the owners of sex establishments rather than the individual sex workers (Kerrigan et al., 2006).

Finally, it is worth bearing in mind that in 'concentrated HIV epidemics' (those in which HIV is mainly limited to groups with higher risk behaviour), interventions targeting sex workers may need to be strategic, concerned with reducing onward transmission as well as sex workers' health.

The most effective interventions promoting health in commercial sex may be those that work at a structural level *and* put sex workers in a position that increases their negotiating power and their ability to demand and access quality services. New Zealand, which legalized sex work in 2003 and regulates it as it does any other industry, reports positive outcomes for sexual health, and no increase in prostitution (Laverack and Whipple, 2010).

Summary

Sex work is a diverse field. People of all genders sell sex, and they do so in very different settings, even within a single country. The values underlying a society's approach to sex work can have a profound impact on the physical, social, and economic wellbeing of people who sell sex.

Programmes that aim to promote the health of sex workers are currently disproportionately focused on condom promotion and STI treatment. These programmes have shown good results in many countries, especially where public health programmes have worked together with the structures that govern the sex industry. However, the occupational health needs of sex workers go beyond direct sexual health needs, and may include mental health and addiction services. There is a strong public health rationale for working towards legal frameworks that eliminate the criminalization of sex work and reduce the risk of violence, but successful efforts will always depend on decision-makers outside the health field.

Notes

1 Based on the author's analysis of national or regional behavioural surveillance data from Bangladesh, China, India, and Indonesia. For replication of analysis, the Indonesian data and associated code books, go online at http://www.ternyata.org/data-sharing/dataverse/.
2 Based on surveillance reports from Cambodia, China, India, Nepal, Suriname, and Thailand.

References

Campbell C and Cornish F (2010) Towards a 'fourth generation' of approaches to HIV/AIDS management: creating contexts for effective community mobilization, *AIDS Care: Psychological and Socio-medical Aspects of AIDS/HIV*, 22: 1569–79.

Celentano DD, Nelson KE, Lyles CM, Beyrer C, Eiumtrakul S, Go VF et al. (1998) Decreasing incidence of HIV and sexually transmitted diseases in young Thai men: evidence for success of the HIV/AIDS control and prevention program, *AIDS*, 12(5): F29–F36.

Chapkis W (2011) Sex workers: interview with Wendy Chapkis, in S. Seidman, N Fischer and C Meeks (eds.) *Introducing the New Sexuality Studies*. Abingdon: Routledge.

Cusick L (2006) Widening the harm reduction agenda: from drug use to sex work, *International Journal of Drug Policy*, 17: 3–11.

Davies N (2009) Inquiry fails to find single trafficker who forced anybody into prostitution, *The Guardian*, 20 October. Available at: http://www.guardian.co.uk/uk/2009/oct/20/government-trafficking-enquiry-fails. Sex work and risk of HIV: male partners of female prostitutes.

Evans C, Jana S and Lambert H (2009) What makes a structural intervention? Reducing vulnerability to HIV in community settings, with particular reference to sex work, *Global Public Health*, 5(5): 449–61.

Hammond N (2010) Tackling taboos: men who pay for sex and the emotional researcher, in K Hardy, S Kingston and T Sanders (eds.) *New Sociologies of Sex Work*. Farnham: Ashgate.

Inciardi JA and Surratt HL (2001) Drug use, street crime and sex trading among cocaine-dependent women: implications for public health and criminal justice policy, *Journal of Psychoactive Drugs*, 33: 379–89.

Jana S, Basu I, Rotheram-Borus MJ and Newman PA (2004) The Sonagachi Project: a sustainable community intervention program, *AIDS Education and Prevention*, 16(5): 405–14.

Kerrigan, D, Moreno L, Rosario S, Gomez B, Jerez H, Barrington C et al. (2006) Environmental-structural interventions to reduce HIV/STI risk among female sex workers in the Dominican Republic, *American Journal of Public Health*, 96(1): 120–5.

Laverack G and Whipple A (2010) The sirens' song of empowerment: a case study of health promotion and the New Zealand Prostitutes Collective, *Global Health Promotion*, 17(1): 33–8.

Lowndes CM, Alary M and Platt L (2003) Injection drug use, commercial sex work, and the HIV/STI epidemic in the Russian Federation, *Sexually Transmitted Diseases*, 30(1): 46–8.

Ministry of Health, Republic of Indonesia (2009) *Estimasi Populasi Dewasa Rawan Terinfeksi HIV 2009*. Jakarta.

Monitoring the AIDS Pandemic (2004) *AIDS in Asia: Face the Facts*. MAP Network.

Pickering H, Todd J, Dunn D, Pepin J and Wilkins A (1992) Prostitutes and their clients: a Gambian survey, *Social Science and Medicine*, 34(1): 75–88.

Pisani E 2008. *The Wisdom of Whores: Bureaucrats, Brothels and the Business of AIDS*. London: Granta Books.

Plumridge L and Abel G (2001) A 'segmented' sex industry in New Zealand: sexual and personal safety of female sex workers, *Australian and New Zealand Journal of Public Health*, 225: 78–83.

Sanders T (2008) *Paying for Pleasure: Men who Buy Sex*. Cullompton: Willan Publishing.

Scambler G and Paoli F (2008) Health work, female sex workers and HIV/AIDS: global and local dimensions of stigma and deviance as barriers to effective interventions, *Social Science and Medicine*, 66(8): 1848–62.

Mobile populations

9

Joanna Busza

Overview

In this chapter, we explore the relationship between the movement of people and their sexual health. First, we describe the different types of geographical migration and their association with sexual behaviour, health outcomes and use of services. Next, we explore the reasons why migrants may experience increased vulnerability, and consider how migrating people's background characteristics, motivations for travel and new environments interact to shape their sexual health. We also introduce strategies to address mobility-related health issues, including targeted policy and interventions.

Learning outcomes

After reading this chapter, you will be able to:

- Identify different types of population movement and their characteristics
- Understand ways in which migration and travel can influence sexual behaviour and health outcomes
- Critique policy and programme approaches that have been used to prevent or mitigate sexual health risks associated with mobility

Key terms

Host population: Pre-existing residents of a country or region into which large numbers of migrants settle, whose own health and behaviour may be influenced by the arrival of new socio-cultural groups.

Migration: General demographic term encompassing long-term resettlement involving *emigration* from one country and *immigration* to another, *cyclical migration* comprising several return trips often for seasonal or temporary work, and *forced migration* (i.e. to avoid conflict or natural disasters).

Mobility: Any form of geographical movement by individuals, communities or whole populations, over short or long distances, within or across national or regional boundaries.

Tourism: Shorter-term travel, often for leisure, although sometimes combined with work or education. Increasingly, *health tourism* refers to travel where the explicit intention is to obtain medical services overseas that are perceived to be less expensive, of higher quality or more easily obtained than in the country of origin.

Introduction

People travel for all sorts of reasons: as tourists to experience new places and cultures, as job-seekers hoping to find better work or higher pay, as immigrants to set up home in a new country, or as refugees fleeing war, political persecution or catastrophic events. At the individual level, when a person moves from one setting to another, he or she is exposed to a different health environment – new infectious diseases, unfamiliar behavioural norms, and services or medicines dissimilar to those found at home. At population level, migration brings mobile groups and host populations into contact with each other, producing change in their health profiles, expectations, and needs. While this is true for many health conditions, it is particularly important for sexual health because so many of its determinants (risk-taking behaviour, social marginalization, poor access to prevention and treatment) can be closely associated with migration.

Sexual health on the move: what is the evidence?

Early in the study of the HIV epidemic, researchers noticed that individuals reporting frequent or long-term travel in surveys also had a higher likelihood of being HIV positive (Decosas et al., 1995). Particularly in East and Southern Africa, the HIV epidemic followed the movement of people across transportation and labour routes, first between urban settings and then from urban to rural environments (Glynn et al., 2001; Lagarde et al., 2003). In many countries around the world, HIV rates are higher among migrants than in the general population, either because the migrants come from places with higher HIV prevalence to start with, or because they engage in higher risk behaviour. In the UK, for instance, about 70% of all HIV diagnoses occur among people born outside the UK, the vast majority of whom are likely to have acquired the infection abroad (Mayor, 2006). In addition, higher HIV rates are found among Burmese men working in the fishing industry in Thailand, a trend linked to their alcohol consumption and lack of condom use with Thai sex workers (Ford and Chamratrithirong, 2008).

Migrants have also been found to be at increased risk of other sexual health problems, including poor pregnancy outcomes, sexual violence, and sexually transmitted infections (STIs). A systematic review of studies across Western Europe found immigrant women had significantly higher risk of having low birth weight babies, premature delivery, and perinatal mortality (Bollini et al., 2007). In research from China, the prevalence of *Chlamydia* was three times higher in women migrating from rural to urban areas (Wang et al., 2010).

Yet the association between mobility and poorer sexual health is by no means universal; indeed, the 'healthy migrant effect' – where migrants demonstrate better health than the host population – has long been acknowledged. This occurs when the healthiest individuals are the ones to leave their homes and relocate, or when communities bring safer sexual practices or treatment-seeking behaviour from their place of origin. For example, in Mexico, sex workers who migrated from rural areas into the city of Tijuana were more likely to register with health services and had significantly lower STI rates than those who were local (Ojeda et al., 2009). In other settings, research has found no difference in sexual health outcomes by migration status, such as analysis of a nationally representative sample of Indian men in which neither STI prevalence nor risk behaviour was associated with long-term or temporary mobility (Gupta et al., 2010).

Activity 9.1

As mentioned above, some studies have unexpectedly found that migrant sex workers have lower STI rates and higher rates of condom use than those from the local area. What factors might explain this and what additional information is needed?

Feedback

To explain the unexpected protectiveness of migration in these settings, one would need to learn more about the wider context of sex work and demographic profiles of the sex workers. Migrant women who initiate sex work may be very different kinds of people from local sex workers. They might differ by age, economic class or ethnic background, all of which would affect their pre-existing health status, confidence in negotiating condom use, and motivation to use services. It is also possible that migrant and local sex workers work in different establishments, which themselves are associated with different levels of risk (working indoors in bars, clubs or hotels is often safer than street-based sex work) or see different types of clients.

Thus the relationship between migration and sexual health is not straightforward. It reflects heterogeneity in experiences of migration, as well as differences in gender, class, and ethnicity between migrant groups. It is therefore crucial to understand the wider context of mobility: *who* is moving, *why* they are doing so, and *how* do they interact with their new environment.

Pathways to risk: what makes migrants vulnerable?

One way to classify migrants is by the motivations behind their decision to move. Conceptual frameworks about migration often refer to 'push' and 'pull' factors as well as more 'upstream' or structural determinants.

Activity 9.2

What might influence individuals or groups in deciding to leave their homes and travel elsewhere for short or long periods of time? How might these factors lead to different health outcomes?

Feedback

'Push' factors occur in people's original place of residence and catalyse their decision to leave, such as poverty, family dissolution or personal misfortune, environmental disasters, and political conflict. These can occur at the individual level (for instance, moving away from home following a relationship break-up) or affect whole communities (e.g. a political conflict or environmental disaster occurs, making a whole region unsafe to live in). 'Pull' factors provide a positive incentive to travel elsewhere, including better wages or living conditions, educational opportunities, asylum from persecution or wanting to see new places. The particular combination of reasons for travel will determine whether people can control what happens to them, how they perceive their situation, and what new risks and opportunities they face. In turn, these experiences influence health behaviour and care.

Why people travel

Travelling for recreation

Tourism as a leisure activity has grown over the years with the ease of international travel, and over 800 million people per year travel for reasons other than work. Tourism takes people away from daily routines and social restrictions, and is often associated in their minds with adventure, pleasure, relaxation, and the opportunity to try new experiences. As a result, tourists may experiment with new sexual behaviours or take more risks. The term 'sex tourism' has been coined to refer to travel for the explicit purpose of engaging in new, different or multiple sexual experiences. Use of alcohol or other intoxicating substances is associated with both holiday travel and unprotected sex.

In a survey of British backpackers to Australia, travellers reported an increase in number of sexual partners while away, inconsistent (40.9%) or no condom use (24.0%) with multiple partners, with consumption of alcohol or illicit drugs among the indicators of risk (Hughes et al., 2009). On a larger scale, a national probability sample of 12,110 British men and women aged 16–44 years found 14% of men and 7% of women reported acquiring at least one new sexual partner while abroad in the five years before the survey (Mercer et al., 2007).

Tourism is also a way for long-term migrants to visit family and friends in their home countries, maintaining contact with their cultures of origin. Where people have moved from regions with higher prevalence of sexual health problems to those with lower prevalence, return trips home can put the migrants at risk and could make them a potential 'bridging population' to others in the country of residence (Xiridou et al., 2010). This will depend on migrants' patterns of sexual behaviour and networking in both locations, and is difficult to assess given the ambiguity surrounding where infections have been acquired.

Finally, the concept of 'health tourism' has been introduced to describe travel for the explicit purpose of obtaining treatment when it is more readily available or cheaper than in the home country. Some countries, including Thailand and South Africa, market themselves internationally as providing high-quality medical services at reasonable costs. Services for international clients are usually provided in elite, private hospitals and are thus available primarily to the wealthy and may draw resources away from more equitable health provision.

Expanding livelihood opportunities

Labour migration occurs legally and illegally, within country boundaries and internationally, for long-term relocation or short-term business trips. The literature on why people who move for economic reasons can experience poorer sexual health is vast, but tends to focus on two issues: (1) exposure to risk during travel and in new environments and (2) limited access to preventive and treatment services.

In terms of behavioural risk, a combination of loneliness, opportunity, the need to alleviate stress, and peer pressure leads some migrants to participate in higher risk sexual activities. 'Cyclical' or 'circular' labour migration describes movement for extended periods of time with fairly regular return trips home. This separates families and can increase the chance that spouses will forge new sexual relationships. Many studies exploring links between migration and HIV in sub-Saharan Africa have highlighted the role of these migrant men in the epidemic. Reports of multiple sexual relationships while away led to the assumption that home communities were subsequently placed at risk since it would be unlikely that married couples would negotiate condom use when reunited; more recently, however, research on women left behind in home communities has shown that they are also likely to engage in higher risk sex during the separation, and transmit HIV to their returning partner (Lurie et al., 2003). This demonstrates the role gender can play in the interaction between sexual health and labour migration.

Activity 9.3

In what ways might the sexual health problems faced by male and female migrants differ?

Feedback

Work opportunities are often different for men and women, so whole workforces may comprise a single sex. Concentrations of mobile men in industries such as transport, industrial-scale agriculture, and mining (i.e. for oil, minerals, precious metals or gems) create risk environments for the spread of STIs and HIV, characterized by consumption of alcohol, multiple sexual partnerships, commercial sex, and low use of condoms in settings as diverse as South Africa (Campbell, 2000) and Canada (Goldenberg et al., 2008). Women who migrate into 'feminized' jobs (such as domestic service or factory work) often face sexual harassment, or are unable to support themselves without supplementing their incomes through transactional sex. In-depth studies of sexual behaviour among young migrant workers in garment factories in Cambodia and Nepal found that poor wages, harsh treatment by factory managers (including sexual advances), and restricted socio-economic opportunities led women into high-risk sexual encounters and limited their ability to request condom use (Nishigaya, 2002; Puri and Busza, 2004; Puri and Cleland, 2007).

Reducing risk

When migrants do experience sexual health risks or problems, they often have limited access to care. This can be because they do not know where to go, have no free time, do not speak the local language or because they are ineligible to use local health facilities. Stigma surrounding sexual behaviour will also discourage the use of specialized services if migrants are part of a small or tight-knit community and do not want to be recognized. Migrants may also fear they will be mistreated or poorly understood by health professionals from different ethnic backgrounds or cultures.

A particularly important distinction among labour migrants is between those who have legal status and those who are undocumented. The former group are better able to reduce their vulnerability and find requisite care, while those without formal status will not only have difficulties in protecting themselves or seeking treatment, but may also find themselves in situations that exacerbate sexual health risks. Where there are no legal routes into existing job opportunities, individuals are more likely to be exploited by people smugglers or traffickers.

Finally, it is worth mentioning the role that migration of *health professionals* has in shaping sexual health, particularly in terms of its impact on services in 'sending' countries. Researchers have suggested that high rates of maternal morbidity and mortality in some select developing countries are partly a result of the loss of sexual and reproductive health personnel, pointing out that up to 25% of doctors and 40% of nurses in the USA have been trained abroad, the majority in low- or middle-income countries (Serour, 2009). As health professionals migrate for the same diversity of reasons as other mobile groups, they may not be easily incentivized to remain in their country of origin.

Displacement

At the end of 2009, UNHCR estimated there were 10.4 million refugees and 15.6 million internally displaced people around the world (Zimmerman et al., 2011). People fleeing conflict or political repression may end up in dangerous and unstable environments and sexual violence and rape often make up the experience of conflict. Some refugees live in organized camps while others are dispersed in urban slums, with little or no access to basic infrastructure or services including health care. As a result, refugees can have poorer sexual and reproductive health than the host population (Busza and Lush, 1999; Wayte et al., 2008). Documented examples record high STI rates, unmet need for contraception and safe abortion, and adverse pregnancy outcomes in refugee populations (Vangen et al., 2008; Benner et al., 2010).

The categories of migrants discussed above are not mutually exclusive, and individual circumstances evolve over time. Someone may start out as a tourist, but then decide to extend their stay by working in a foreign country and eventually settle there permanently. Cyclical migrants might also find they return home less and less frequently, and set up residence where they have steady work. On the other hand, descendents from refugee groups born away from their family's country of origin sometimes continue to consider themselves to be forced migrants and do not wish to, or are prevented from, integrating into the host population.

Catching up: how can health systems meet the needs of mobile populations?

The development of policies and programmes to address migrants' sexual health clearly need to consider mobile populations as a dynamic group, who not only represent a wide range of migration experiences but who will also change in composition over time, with concomitant changes in their health and needs.

Identifying migrants can present significant challenges, particularly if they do not have legal status, are widely dispersed or do not want to attract the attention of the authorities. In some cases, migrants are concentrated in occupations that are illegal or stigmatized (such as sex work), so are unwilling to attend health facilities, even if they are eligible. In these cases, separating public health from law enforcement is critical to ensure a rights-based approach to health. Arrangements can be made with police to guarantee that no adverse consequences result from undocumented migrants' use of harm reduction or medical services. Regular contact with key informants (such as community leaders) is also important to keep abreast of the arrival and movement of new waves of migrants.

Furthermore, physical and social barriers to access of services may need special efforts to overcome. On a practical level, transportation may be difficult to find or prohibitively expensive, or clinics may not be open at times convenient for migrants, particularly if they work long or irregular hours. Mobile or outreach services can provide basic care or referrals to migrants where they live and work, or 'drop in' clinics can be established that are located in convenient sites and open at times migrants are available, for example, late in the evenings at the end of work shifts.

Language or cultural beliefs also affect use of services, and hiring staff from the target community will make clients feel more comfortable. Where there is a mix of nationalities, services can use interpreters to translate client–provider interactions as required. Ideally, interpreters provide insight into migrants' health beliefs, traditional practices, and likely concerns in addition to translating conversations. Engaging community members in promoting health messages, disseminating information about available services, and helping to ensure facilities are 'migrant friendly' will further improve programme effectiveness and sustainability.

Activity 9.4

About half of the world's refugees are now classified as 'urban' refugees, meaning they are dispersed in large cities and settlements, rather than housed in organized refugee camps. What are the implications for delivering sexual health services to them?

Feedback

Because urban refugees are scattered throughout concentrated settlements, often slum areas, they can be difficult to identify among the rest of the host population, particularly if from the same ethnic or cultural background. Furthermore, urban refugees are less likely to be formally recognized or given documentation by agencies such as the UN Agency for Refugees (UNHCR), so may be perceived locally as illegal migrants who are ineligible for care. The challenges of providing services will mirror those for other types of migrants in marginalized settings with over-stretched health systems. There are also ethical issues related to targeting refugees over the rest of the population, who may also have poor access. However, refugees might have special needs related to their experiences of violence, trauma, and conflict before and during transit. Using peer-to-peer approaches, locating services close to concentrations of refugees, and ensuring services are culturally acceptable, open at convenient times, and free will help to identify and attract migrants in need of care.

Summary

The category of mobile populations encompasses people with a wide diversity of travel experiences. People move for a complex mix of reasons, and encounter new situations over which they have varying degrees of control. While not all mobile populations experience greater threats to their sexual health, considerable international evidence exists suggesting that for many, both short- and long-term travel can enhance migrants' vulnerability. Negotiating movement across unfamiliar geographical terrain and in new cultural contexts is often associated with increases in sexual risk behaviour and decreased access to prevention and treatment services. Illegal status, forced migration, and marginalized living conditions will exacerbate the determinants of vulnerability, while strong social ties, better socio-economic position, and targeted services that aim to reach the most 'hidden' populations will mitigate these. Ultimately, understanding the background, motivations, and context of mobile populations is critical for responding effectively to their sexual health needs.

References

Benner MT, Townsend J, Kaloi W, Htwe K, Naranichakul N, Hunnangkul S et al. (2010) Reproductive health and quality of life of young Burmese refugees in Thailand, *Conflict and Health*, 4(5).

Bollini P, Stotzer U and Wanner P (2007) Pregnancy outcomes and migration in Switzerland: results from a focus group study, *International Journal of Public Health*, 52(2): 78–86.

Busza J and Lush L (1999) Planning reproductive health in conflict: a conceptual framework, *Social Science and Medicine*, 49(2): 155–71.

Campbell C (2000) Selling sex in the time of AIDS: the psycho-social context of condom use by sex workers on a Southern African mine, *Social Science and Medicine*, 50: 479–94.

Decosas J, Kane F, Anarfi JK, Sodji KD and Wagner HU (1995) Migration and AIDS, *Lancet*, 346(8978): 826–8.

Ford K and Chamratrithirong A (2008) Migrant seafarers and HIV risk in Thai communities, *AIDS Education and Prevention*, 20(5): 454–63.

Glynn JR, Pönnighaus J, Crampin AC, Sibande F, Sichali L, Nkhosa P et al. (2001) The development of the HIV epidemic in Karonga District, Malawi, *AIDS*, 15(15): 2025–9.

Goldenberg SM, Shoveller JA, Ostry AC and Koehoorn M (2008) Sexually transmitted infection (STI) testing among young oil and gas workers: the need for innovative, place-based approaches to STI control, *Canadian Journal of Public Health*, 99(4): 350–4.

Gupta K, Vaidehi Y and Majumder N (2010) Spatial mobility, alcohol use, sexual behavior and sexual health among males in India, *AIDS and Behavior*, 14(suppl. 1): 18–30.

Hughes K, Downing J, Bellis MA, Dillon P and Copeland J (2009) The sexual behaviour of British backpackers in Australia, *Sexually Transmitted Infections*, 85(6): 477–82.

Lagarde E, Schim van der Loeff M, Enel C, Holmgren B, Dray-Spira R, Pison G et al. (2003) Mobility and the spread of human immunodeficiency virus into rural areas of West Africa, *International Journal of Epidemiology*, 32(5): 744–52.

Lurie MN, Williams BG, Zuma K, Mkaya-Mwamburi D, Garnett GP, Sweat MD et al. (2003) Who infects whom? HIV-1 concordance and discordance among migrant and non-migrant couples in South Africa, *AIDS*, 17(15): 2245–52.

Mayor S (2006) Report on health of migrants to UK shows high risk of TB and HIV, *British Medical Journal*, 333(7578): 1088.

Mercer CH, Fenton KA, Wellings K, Copas AJ, Erens B and Johnson AM (2007) Sex partner acquisition while overseas: results from a British national probability survey, *Sexually Transmitted Infections*, 83(7): 517–22.

Nishigaya K (2002) Female garment factory workers in Cambodia: migration, sex work and HIV/AIDS, *Women and Health*, 35(4): 27–42.

Ojeda V, Strathdee SA, Lozada R, Rusch ML, Fraga M, Orozovich P et al. (2009) Associations between migrant status and sexually transmitted infections among female sex workers in Tijuana, Mexico, *Sexually Transmitted Infections*, 85(6): 420–6.

Puri M and Busza J (2004) In forests and factories: sexual behaviour among young migrant workers in Nepal, *Culture, Health and Sexuality*, 6(2): 145–58.

Puri M and Cleland J (2007) Assessing the factors associated with sexual harassment among young female migrant workers in Nepal, *Journal of Interpersonal Violence*, 22(11): 1363–81.

Serour GI (2009) Healthcare workers and the brain drain, *International Journal of Gynecology and Obstetrics*, 106(2): 175–8.

Vangen S, Eskild A and Forsen L (2008) Termination of pregnancy according to immigration status: a population-based registry linkage study, *British Journal of Obstetrics and Gynaecology*, 115(10): 1309–15.

Wang W, Wei C, Buchholz ME, Martin MC, Smith BD, Huang ZJ et al. (2010) Prevalence and risks for sexually transmitted infections among a national sample of migrants versus non-migrants in China, *International Journal of STD and AIDS*, 21(6): 410–15.

Wayte K, Zwi AB, Belton S, Martins J, Martins N, Whelan A et al. (2008) Conflict and development: challenges in responding to sexual and reproductive health needs in Timor-Leste, *Reproductive Health Matters*, 16(31): 83–92.

Xiridou M, van Veen M, Coutinho R and Prins M (2010) Can migrants from high-endemic countries cause new HIV outbreaks among heterosexuals in low-endemic countries?, *AIDS*, 24(13): 2081–8.

Zimmerman C, Kiss L and Hossain M (2011) Migration and health: a framework for 21st century policy-making, *PLoS Medicine*, 8(5): e1001034.

Further reading

Augustin LM (2007) *Sex at the Margins: Migration, Labour Markets and the Rescue Industry*. London: Zed Books.

Deane KD, Parkhurst JO and Johnston D (2010) Linking migration, mobility and HIV, *Tropical Medicine and International Health*, 15(12): 1458–63.

Gardner R and Blackburn R (1996) People who move: new reproductive health focus, *Population Reports*, Series J(45): 1–27.

Gushulak B and MacPherson D (2006) The basic principles of migration health: population mobility and gaps in disease prevalence, *Emerging Themes in Epidemiology*, 3(1): 3.

International Organization for Migration (undated) Various resources available at: www.iom.int.

Minimum Initial Services Package for Reproductive Health in Crisis Situation (MISP). Available at: http://misp.rhrc.org/. Provides information on a global initiative to provide reproductive and sexual health services to refugee populations.

Zimmerman C, Kiss L and Hossain M (2011) Migration and health: a framework for 21st century policy-making, *PLoS Medicine*, 8(5): e1001034.

10 Structural influences on sexual health

Martine Collumbien, Jessica Datta, Benjamin Davis and Kaye Wellings

Overview

In this chapter, we focus on features of the social, economic, and political environment that influence vulnerability and risk. Interest in addressing the structural drivers of sexual health has increased with recognition of the limited success of public health interventions focusing narrowly on individual risk behaviour. We examine the relationship between structural factors and sexual health status, and the mechanisms that help explain this relationship. We trace the pathways through which they operate and the interaction between the multiple influences. Finally, we identify the consequences for sexual health policy and practice.

Learning outcomes

After reading this chapter, you will be able to:

- Identify structural factors and understand their importance in shaping vulnerability and risk
- Gain insight into the relationships between sexual health status, poverty, gender and their interplay with other structural factors
- Understand the need for a focus on social structural factors in sexual health policy and programming

Key terms

Risk: The likelihood that an individual is exposed to an adverse sexual health outcome (such as sexually transmitted infection (STI), unplanned pregnancy, dysfunction or sexual violence).

Vulnerability: Extent of exposure to ill health stemming from social contextual factors that are largely exogenous – that is, beyond the control of individual agency.

Introduction

As noted in earlier chapters, the wide variation between and within populations underlines the powerful role of social contextual factors in shaping sexual behaviour and sexual health status. An increasing public health focus on the role of broader structural factors in explaining sexual health differentials has been prompted by the absence of a strong and consistent association between sexual behaviour and sexual health outcomes (Buvé and Bishikwabo-Nsarhaza, 2002; Wellings et al., 2006), and by evidence from evaluation studies of the limited impact of sexual health interventions that simply address individual risk behaviour and ignore broader structural factors (Coates et al., 2008; Padian et al., 2010).

What do we mean by structural factors?

At the heart of a social structural perspective is the recognition that behaviour is more than merely a personal choice. Social structures, institutions, and norms provide the potential for, and impose limitations on, human agency and action. The notion of the 'duality' of agency and structure, such that we act *upon* but also *within* the world we inhabit, helps to frame the distinction between individual risk behaviours and social structural factors (Giddens, 1979).

This theme has been extensively explored in the political economy of health model of public health. Central to this model is the recognition that factors external to the individual, such as inequitable power structures, absolute and relative poverty and differential access to resources, social isolation and discrimination restrict an individual's ability to achieve positive health outcomes or to facilitate change. These factors create 'risk environments' that disproportionately influence the health outcomes of the poorest and the most vulnerable.

Several attempts have been made to provide a conceptual framework within which structural factors can be set. Most have tried to characterize structural influences by the level at which they operate, distinguishing between distal and proximate factors in the causal pathway to individual action.

Operating at a greater distance from individual action are macro-level factors such as the national and global economy, levels of development, political organization and systems of governance, and social norms often underpinned by laws. Public policies are included in macro-level influences, which encompass provision of education and healthcare services, transport, and housing. Distal factors also include transitions associated with political change and conflict in a region, and socio-economic and demographic trends such as urbanization and migration.

At a more proximate level, community-based inequalities foster differentials in sexual health status. They include inequalities in wealth, income and availability of resources, relative and absolute area-level deprivation, population density, adequacy of transport systems and access to public health interventions and healthcare facilities, and social organizational factors such as social cohesion.

In the more immediate context of the lives of individuals, living conditions, personal relationships, and financial resources have the potential to influence health. Area of residence (urban or rural) and educational level are also associated with risk and vulnerability, as are less easily measured factors such as social capital (the degree to which lives are connected in a supportive and health-enhancing way). Individual-level factors affect resilience to the impact of macro-level environmental factors.

The influence of structural factors may be direct and concrete, for example, where inability to afford condoms and other contraception supplies results in unprotected sex. Alternatively, it may be indirect and less obvious. The perpetration of sexual violence without shame or remorse, or failure to heed safer sex messages or to respect the sexual autonomy of an individual, may appear to be the result of personal decision-making, but may in fact reflect powerful social norms in a community of which individuals are unaware.

A useful framework with which to understand the different levels at which structural influences operate draws on an ecological model of behaviour that situates individuals in a nested set of increasing social circles, illustrated in Figure 10.1.

Identifying structural influences

A major structural influence on health status is poverty, both in its absolute form and its relative form, inequality. Poverty can be operationalized in many different ways, but most definitions recognize that human development goes beyond purely economic factors. Broader definitions embrace concepts such as participation, citizenship, and capability (Sen, 1992).

Asset-poor countries are restricted in terms of the resources that can be made available for educational and sexual health service interventions, and economic adversity restricts the power of men and women to take control of their sexual health. At the individual level, poorer members of societies may lack the means to adopt risk reduction strategies and to make use of healthcare provision. And where more pressing concerns relate to basic survival and earning a livelihood, sexual health may be deemed a low priority.

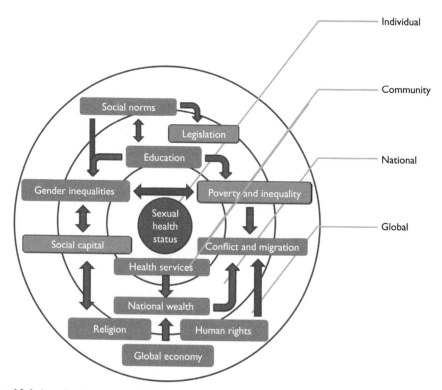

Figure 10.1 Levels of structural influences on sexual health

The link between poverty and sexual health is complicated by the multiplicity of interacting social and contextual factors. Gender, geographical location (urban or rural), and educational level are also associated with risk and vulnerability, as are social factors, which are less easy to measure, such as sexual networks, social capital, community resilience, and gender inequality.

Gender interacts especially powerfully with poverty and deprivation to create vulnerability. As we saw in earlier chapters, while the term 'sex' refers to the biological and physiological characteristics that define men and women, gender refers to the socially constructed roles, behaviours, activities, and attributes that a given society considers appropriate for men and women. The effect of poverty is inextricably linked to gender, to women's status, and the socially defined roles of women in many societies. Gendered divisions of labour may limit women's ability to enter the workplace and their control over resources. Gendered power imbalances may limit potential for negotiation for safer sex, and even the ability to access health services, particularly where there is financial dependency or the threat of violence.

Social norms relating to gender, age, and sexual diversity are also potent structural influences on sexual health. The sexual double standard, whereby restraint is expected of women, whereas excesses are tolerated for men, hinders attempts by men and women to protect their sexual health. Non-exclusive sexual relationships are more likely to be condoned for men, and may even be encouraged. The importance of gender norms for sexual health outcomes has long been recognized, and the HIV epidemic brought gender into even sharper focus. Yet attention has also been paid recently to ways in which gender norms impact on men's lives. Many stereotypically 'masculine' traits – a reluctance to express vulnerability or seek help, excessive alcohol use, having multiple sexual partners – are at odds with the protection and maintenance of sexual health.

Economic, social, and political transitions also affect sexual health status, particularly where they give rise to inequalities or social dislocation. In earlier chapters, we discussed the link between social disruption associated with conflict and sexual violence and transactional sex. The link has also been drawn between abrupt political change and injecting drug use, the main risk factor for HIV in Russia (Rhodes et al., 2005) (see below).

Structural factors and sexual health: the evidence for the relationship

Evidence for the influence of structural factors on sexual health status is drawn from several sources. At the macro level, ecological analyses (i.e. from comparative analyses of indicators of levels of wealth and sexual health status at national level) have found correlations between adverse sexual health outcomes and a range of material indicators, including poverty, wealth, income inequality, and national income. At the micro level, focusing on individuals or households, the evidence linking poverty, gender, and other structural factors with poor sexual health outcomes such as STIs, unwanted births, unsafe abortion, and access to contraception comes largely from retrospective cross-sectional studies, such as the World Fertility Surveys and the Demographic and Health Surveys. It also comes from qualitative research examining the processes by which social contextual factors increase risk for particular groups (e.g. young women, truck drivers, sex workers) or outcomes (e.g. gender-based violence, migration, and unprotected sex).

The evidence for a link between socio-economic status and adverse reproductive health outcomes is fairly unequivocal. At a global level, women living in low- and middle-income countries experience higher levels of morbidity and mortality attributed to sexual and reproductive health than do women in wealthier countries. A study of modern contraceptive use in 55 developing countries found a consistent and increasing gap between rich and poor in the use of modern contraception, within and between countries (Gakidou and Vayena, 2007). Education is a powerful mediator in this context; an extensive literature is devoted to the role of education in sustaining fertility control (Channon et al., 2010). As we saw in Chapter 3, the likelihood of having an abortion is roughly similar for women in rich and poor countries, but women from poor countries are far more likely to die as a result of an unsafe abortion.

Inequality is also associated with poorer sexual health. The prevalence of adverse sexual health outcomes is higher in countries in which there are wide discrepancies in income distribution, and this has been attributed to health inequalities being associated with lower levels of trust and weaker social capital (Wilkinson, 2005: 63). Teenage births provide an example of this relationship. In high-income countries such as the UK and USA, which have wider inequalities in income, teenage birth rates are higher than in countries with more equal income distribution (Wilkinson and Pickett, 2010).

The impact of STIs on quality and length of life also varies with national levels of wealth. More than 90% of the global disability-adjusted life years (DALY) caused by STIs, excluding HIV, are experienced in low- and middle-income countries and over 50% of the global burden is suffered by women in low-income countries (Chapter 2).

More than 60% of people living with HIV live in the world's poorest region, sub-Saharan Africa. Within regions, however, there are inconsistencies in this broad general pattern. In sub-Saharan Africa, it is the middle ranking countries in terms of wealth, as well as those with greater income inequality, that are most affected by HIV (Piot et al., 2007). The evidence at individual level is also equivocal. A systematic review found that in east, central, and southern Africa, women with a higher income and educational level were at increased risk of HIV (Wojcicki, 2005). Findings such as these have prompted the observation that 'both wealth and poverty may have associated risks and protective effects in different contexts' (Parkhurst, 2010). As the African AIDS epidemic matures, the key drivers may be not poverty itself, but economic and gender inequalities and weakened social ties in communities associated with rapid growth (Piot et al., 2007). AIDS is now seen as a disease associated with economic transition, rather than a disease of poverty in itself (Piot et al., 2007).

Evidence of the impact of social, economic, and political transitions on sexual health is available from other settings. In the decade after political transition, Russia saw a 20-fold increase in the number of registered injecting drug users. Expanding transport and communication networks fostered migration and mixing of populations, and economic restructuring weakened public health infrastructures but created local informal economies in which drug and sex markets flourished. Abrupt and rapid change contributed to the weakening of civil society, diminishing social cohesion and creating economic hardship. The geographical distribution of HIV genotypes was found to be consistent with transmission patterns associated with transport, trade, and tourism (Rhodes et al., 2005).

Understanding the causal pathways

Although there is clearly a relationship between structural factors and sexual health status, there are also anomalies and inconsistencies in the evidence base, reflecting the complexity of structural factors and the interplay between them. Identifying the mechanisms explaining the links between structural factors and sexual health is difficult.

Activity 10.1

An understanding of the mechanisms through which poverty, gender, and other structural factors wield an influence on sexual health, and the point at which they operate along the causal pathway to poorer sexual health, is essential to the identification of possible escape routes. But it is nevertheless challenging for a number of reasons. Note down what some of these may be.

Feedback

Structural factors may operate at different points along the causal pathway. One reason for the difficulty in disentangling the effects of structural factors is that they impact differentially at different points along the causal pathway. The risk of any adverse sexual health outcome, for example, depends on the nature and extent of risk behaviours (e.g. early sex or multiple sexual partners); of risk reduction practice (e.g. use of condoms and contraception); and of service use (e.g. preventive or curative prevention or treatment). The influence of structural factors may be harmful at one point, but protective at another. The risk associated with larger numbers of sexual partners among the more socially privileged in some settings might be mitigated by the increased likelihood that sex will be protected and, in the event of unwanted pregnancy or infection, health care will be accessed to obtain emergency contraception, or post-exposure prophylaxis in the case of HIV.

Hallfors and colleagues (2007), for example, found that young black adults in the USA were at risk of STI acquisition even if they reported low levels of sexual risk-taking, while white young adults were only at risk of acquiring an STI if their levels of sexual risk behaviours were high (Hallfors et al., 2007). In rural South Africa, HIV incidence in women was highest in the least educated group, who were no more likely to report multiple sexual partners than the better educated, but were less likely to practise safer sex (Hargreaves et al., 2007).

Structural factors impact differently on different sexual health outcomes. Risk factors vary for different sexual health outcomes. The key risk behaviour for early pregnancy, for example, is early onset of sexual activity, whereas for STIs it is having multiple sexual partners. Structural factors operate differentially on these risk behaviours. Lower levels of educational attainment and higher levels of deprivation are strongly associated with age at onset of sexual activity. The picture is more complex in the case of multiple sexual partnerships. In some settings, these are more common where poverty drives the sale of sex, or where migration associated with the search for employment creates the conditions for non-exclusive relationships. In others, multiple partnerships may be a consequence of a longer time spent in education, delayed marriage or cohabitation, and higher disposable income. The two effects may co-exist in the same population; wealth may enable men to buy sex, but poverty drives women to sell it. This may explain why, in some contexts, HIV/STI prevalence is more weakly associated with poverty *per se* than is reproductive health, or sexual violence.

Structural factors interact differently in different settings. Vulnerability to poor sexual health depends on the interaction between structural factors, and this in turn depends on the context in which they operate. For example, in some settings, living in an urban area may pose a greater risk to sexual health than living in a rural area.

Multiple sexual partnerships may be more common where urban poverty interacts with low levels of social capital; where the anonymity of city life predisposes people to seek intimacy and at the same time shields them from community disapproval; and where there is an absence of social cohesion. In settings in which the infrastructure is weak, where transport links are poor, where resources do not allow adequate coverage in terms of access to sexual health services, living in a rural area may be associated with poorer sexual health.

Cycles of deprivation

The relationship between poverty and sexual health is bi-directional. Just as poverty and gender and other structural factors impact on sexual health, so sexual health impacts on poverty, gender, and even environmental phenomena such as climate change (Green and Merrick, 2005). We can trace several 'vicious spirals' in areas of sexual health. Early childbearing, unplanned pregnancy, and intimate partner and sexual violence are themselves barriers to employment and income generation and risk factors for homelessness, poor self-esteem, and low aspirations (Vyas and Watts, 2009), thus potentially perpetuating the cycle of deprivation.

Activity 10.2

In many developed countries, early pregnancy is more common among women from less well-off backgrounds and with a lower level of educational attainment. Looking at the maps in Figure 10.2, what strikes you about the distribution of teenage pregnancy and the distribution of deprivation in England and Wales? Does what you observe suggest that deprivation leads to teenage pregnancy? Or does teenage pregnancy lead to deprivation? What conclusions do you draw for public health intervention?

Feedback

Unmistakeably, there is a close fit between the highest rates of teenage conceptions and deprivation black spots. Particularly in more developed countries, poverty is a major determinant of early pregnancy. And it is also an outcome of early pregnancy. But is it simply that poverty begets poverty? Do the economic conditions that increased the likelihood of teenage pregnancy simply persist subsequently? The evidence is that although poverty in one generation is repeated in the next, teenage pregnancy adds an extra increment of poverty, so exacerbating pre-existing deprivation. Because of the circular nature of causality, a public health intervention at any point in the cycle has the potential to be effective. This was the premise on which the English government's Teenage Pregnancy Strategy, 2000–2010, was conceived. The dual aims of the strategy were to prevent conception among young people by improving sex education and sexual health services, and to reduce social exclusion among teenage parents by creating opportunities for return to education and employment (Wilkinson et al., 2006).

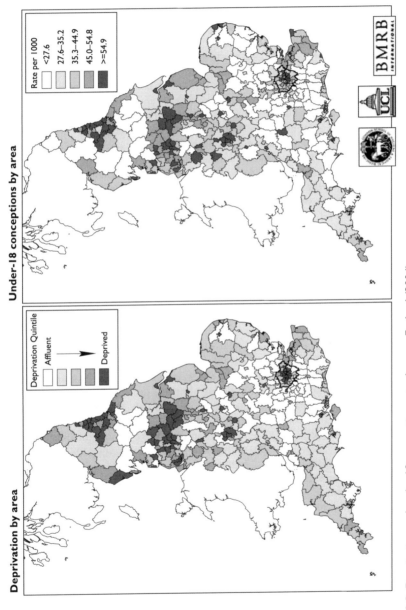

Deprivation by area

Deprivation Quintile

Affluent → Deprived

Under-18 conceptions by area

Rate per 1000
- <27.6
- 27.6–35.2
- 35.3–44.9
- 45.0–54.8
- >=54.9

Figure 10.2 Deprivation and under-18 conception rates by area, England (2004)

Structural interventions in sexual health

Prevention strategies aimed at individual behaviour are likely to change only partially the burden of sexual ill health. Interventions need to be created to create the conditions that support individuals and communities in reducing risk and improving sexual health. Despite recognition of this, sexual health interventions addressing social and contextual factors are still comparatively rare, and those undertaken have met with only limited success (Chapter 12). There remains a gap in both policy and practice around how best to engage with sexual health promotion in a structural way, which goes beyond a focus on individual behaviour change (Rao Gupta et al., 2008).

Structural interventions differ from many public health interventions in that they locate the cause of public health problems in contextual or environmental factors that influence risk behaviour, or other determinants of infection or morbidity, rather than in characteristics of individuals who engage in risk (Blankenship et al., 2006). Individual-focused approaches assume that the relationship between individuals and society is one in which individuals have considerable autonomy to make and act on their choices, but structural approaches view individual agency as constrained or shaped by structures.

A structural approach aims to provide people with the *capacity* to resist sexual health risk within a supportive *environment*. In the context of sexual health, this might include an approach that removes legal, economic or policy obstacles to the adoption by individuals of preventive measures. Examples include creating legal access to free sterile injecting equipment without fear of arrest, making contraception available free of charge, and ensuring that condoms are easily and discretely accessed to reduce fears of social disapproval.

A 'rights-based' approach

Many of the goals relating to structural interventions are beyond the reach of public health agencies and require collaborative, inter-sectoral working supported by political will. At the same time, growing awareness of the complex web of structural factors shaping sexual health risk and vulnerability has prompted a reappraisal of the notion of what constitutes public health practice. The shift is away from seeing public health practice as merely a technical exercise, towards a consideration of its ethical and political dimensions, and its potential as an agent of a broader process of social change and justice (Parker et al., 2004). A human rights framework is valuable in addressing a range of interlocking structural factors, together with legislation that protects human rights (Cáceres et al., 2009; Berer, 2011).

The need to address inequalities in health status, whether borne out of wealth and income differentials, discrimination on the basis of ethnicity or sexual orientation, or power relations contingent on gender or age, has added further impetus to a focus on human rights based approaches to public health in the past two decades. Human rights based approaches are critical in addressing health inequalities and have become cornerstones of all aspects of public health but they are particularly relevant in sexual health.

Rights-based approaches are particularly useful in resolving the tensions that exist between public health and legislative systems. Criminalization of sex work, for example, may encourage police to confiscate condoms from sex workers as proof of illegal practices; laws against homosexuality may make it difficult to convey essential safer sex messages in public education; and legislation relating to the age of sexual consent may impede provision of sexual health services to young people or deter those in need from seeking help from health services. Whether it is a case of criminalization hindering public health efforts, or public health efforts being seen to fall foul of the law, rights-based approaches can help in holding governments and agencies to basic principles safeguarding individual rights with regard to protection and treatment.

Implications for intervention

The breadth and complexity of interventions needed to address structural barriers to sexual health also have implications for evaluation, and the manner in which it is carried out. Interventions that seek to change the more distal factors shaping patterns of sexual behaviour – such as national laws or policies, or programmes that are being delivered on a large scale – such as the AVAHAN HIV prevention programme in Southern India (Chapter 12), lend themselves less well to the application of the randomized trial evaluation model (Chapter 16). An emphasis on structural factors as determinants of sexual health status will also have a bearing on the endpoints used in evaluation of public health interventions. If a key aim of public health programmes is to provide equitable access to services, then decreasing disparities in service utilization will be an important indicator of programme achievement.

Summary

Structural influences on sexual health include a range of social, economic, and political factors operating at a number of levels, from individual action to global policies. The way in which structural factors interact to wield an influence on sexual health status is highly context dependent. Growing evidence on the link between social and structural phenomena and sexual health status affirms the association but also highlights some anomalies. While early pregnancy and intimate partner violence are more clearly associated with socio-economic disadvantage, the relationship between poverty and STIs and HIV shows complex associations at both national and household level. That some studies find correlations between HIV and poverty and others with wealth highlights the context-specific nature of some structural drivers, and the dangers of over-generalization.

The HIV pandemic has taught us much about the importance of socio-cultural, economic, legal, and political contexts in shaping individual risk and health outcomes. Women are more susceptible to adverse sexual health outcomes and the financial dependence of many women, together with gendered expectations of female sexual behaviour and gender roles, further disadvantage women.

Comprehensive multi-level, multi-partner interventions are needed that take account of the social context in mounting individual-level programmes, attempt to modify social norms to support uptake and maintenance of behaviour change, and tackle the structural factors that contribute to risky sexual behaviour. Because the relationship between structural factors and poor sexual outcomes is complex, efforts by public health agencies to address them need to be in collaborative partnership with different sectors and agencies, and supported by political leadership and attention to human rights.

References

Berer M (2011) Repoliticising sexual and reproductive health and rights, *Reproductive Health Matters*, 19(38): 4–10.

Blankenship KM, Friedman SR, Dworkin S and Mantell JE (2006) Structural interventions: concepts, challenges and opportunities for research, *Journal of Urban Health*, 83(1): 59–72.

Buvé A and Bishikwabo-Nsarhaza K (2002) The spread and effect of HIV-1 in sub-Saharan Africa, *Lancet*, 395(9322): 2011–17.

Cáceres CF, Pecheny M, Frasca T, Rios RR and Pocahy F (2009) *Review of Legal Frameworks and the Situation of Human Rights Related to Sexual Diversity in Low and Middle Income Countries*. Geneva: UNAIDS.

Channon AA, Falkingham J and Matthews Z (2010) Sexual and reproductive health and poverty, in S Malarcher (ed.) *Social Determinants of Sexual and Reproductive Health: Informing Future Research and Programme Implementation*. Geneva: WHO.

Coates TJ, Richter L and Cáceres C (2008) Behavioural strategies to reduce HIV transmission: how to make them work better, *Lancet*, 372(9639): 669–84.

Gakidou E and Vayena E (2007) Use of modern contraception by the poor is falling behind, *PLoS Medicine*, 4(2): 381–9.

Giddens A (1979) *Central Problems in Social Theory*. Basingstoke: Macmillan.

Green ME, Merrick T (2005) *Poverty Reduction: Does Reproductive Health Matter?* Washington, DC: International Bank for Reconstruction and Development and The World Bank.

Hallfors DD, Iritani B, Miller WC and Bauer DJ (2007) Sexual and drug behavior patterns and HIV and STD racial disparities: the need for new directions, *American Journal of Public Health*, 97: 125–131.

Hargreaves JR, Bonell CP, Morison LA, Kim JC, Phetla G, Porter JDH et al. (2007) Explaining continued high HIV prevalence in South Africa: socioeconomic factors, HIV incidence and sexual behaviour change among a rural cohort, 2001–2004, *AIDS*, 21(suppl. 7): S39–S48.

Padian NS, McCoy SI, Balkus JE and Wasserheit JN (2010) Weighing the gold in the gold standard: challenges in HIV prevention research, *AIDS*, 24: 621–35.

Parker R, di Mauro D, Filiano B, Garcia J, Muñoz-Laboy M and Sember R (2004) Global transformations and intimate relations in the 21st century: social science research on sexuality and the emergence of sexual health and sexual rights frameworks, *Annual Review of Sex Research*, 15: 362–98.

Parkhurst J (2010) Understanding the correlations between wealth, poverty and human immunodeficiency virus infection in African countries, *Bulletin of the World Health Organization*, 88(7): 519–26.

Piot P, Greener R and Russell S (2007) Squaring the circle: AIDS, poverty, and human development, *PLoS Medicine*, 4(10): 1571–5.

Rao Gupta G, Parkhurst JO, Ogden JA, Aggleton P and Mahal A (2008) Structural approaches to HIV prevention, *Lancet*, 372(9640): 764–75.

Rhodes T, Singer M, Bourgois P, Friedman SR and Strathdee SA (2005) The social structural production of HIV risk among injecting drug users, *Social Science and Medicine*, 61(5): 1026–44.

Sen A (1992) *Inequality Re-examined*. Oxford: Clarendon Press.

Vyas S and Watts C (2009) How does economic empowerment affect women's risk of intimate partner violence in low and middle income countries? A systematic review of published evidence, *Journal of International Development*, 21(5): 577–602.

Wellings K, Collumbien M, Slaymaker E, Singh S, Hodges Z, Patel D et al. (2006) Sexual behaviour in context: a global perspective, *Lancet*, 368: 1706–28.

Wilkinson P, French R, Kane R, Lachowycz K, Stephenson J, Grundy C et al. (2006) Teenage conceptions, abortions, and births in England, 1994–2003, and the national teenage pregnancy strategy, *Lancet*, 368: 1879–86.

Wilkinson RG (2005) *The Impact of Inequality: How to Make Sick Societies Healthier*. London: Routledge.

Wilkinson R and Pickett K (2010) *The Spirit Level: Why Equality is Better for Everyone*. London: Penguin.

Wojcicki JM (2005) Socio-economic status as a risk factor for HIV infection in women in east, central and southern Africa: a systematic review, *Journal of Biosocial Science*, 37: 1–36.

PART 4

Interventions to improve sexual health

Communication and language

11

Kaye Wellings

Overview

Communication is a cornerstone of all areas of sexual health practice, and so is an important theme to tackle before addressing sexual health interventions and research. In this chapter, we explore different ways in which we communicate about sexual matters, the ease with which we are able to do so, and what is allowed expression and what is not. We also reflect on how this varies with social and historical context; and what the particular challenges are for sexual health investigation and intervention.

Learning outcomes

After reading this chapter, you will be able to:

- Understand the significance of modes of communication about sexual matters
- Describe particular challenges for communication about sexual health in the context of research, health promotion, and sexual health services

Key terms

Communication: The transfer of information, including facts, opinions, feelings, and experiences, by verbal and non-verbal means.

Discourse: For linguists, the term 'discourse' is used in the sense of 'language in use'. For critical theorists, 'discourses' are sets of propositions in currency about a particular phenomenon. Both senses are in use in this chapter.

Taboo: A common prohibition based on repression, excluded words, objects, actions or people.

Modes of communication

Despite the title of this chapter, communication does not necessarily involve verbal expression. Speech is but one way – and often not the most important way – of conveying messages about sex. Since sexual behaviour is embodied, it is not surprising that bodily posture, inflections and deflections, and gestures and facial expressions, are powerfully effective modes of sexual expression. So, too, are visual images and objects.

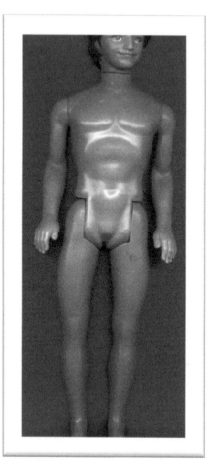

Figure 11.1 Action Man Aladdin: what is missing?

Activity 11.1

Looking at the picture of Aladdin (Figure 11.1), a toy action figure, what messages are conveyed?

Feedback

The fact that Aladdin has no penis sends a powerful message to children that this part of the male anatomy is not for public display. Children learn from an early age what can and cannot be shown or seen in public, and also what cannot be spoken about or heard. Silence, as well as invisibility, conveys meaning. We take many of our cues about sexuality from what can and cannot be given verbal or visual expression.

What is allowed expression?

As discussed in Chapter 1, sexual behaviour is more strongly socially circumscribed than are most other behaviours. Other aspects of human life are subject to taboos – excretion, menstruation, and dying, for example – but they are weaker, and are neither historically nor culturally universal. In ancient Ephesus, for example, the Romans placed public lavatories in the open and adjacent to one another in the town forum, so that the citizens could chat while using them. In general, we tend not to reflect on why some and not other behaviours are permitted expression, so effectively are we socialized into the norms of our society. But it is interesting to test our reactions to hypothetical reversals of these norms, so that repressed subjects are given expression, and vice versa. Such was the aim of Louis Bunuel, in his famous film 'The Discreet Charm of the Bourgeoisie', in which the guests at a dinner party hid behind bushes in the garden to eat and drink, but had open sex at the dinner table.

Language and meaning

Our ideas about sex are closely bound up with language. Language produces the categories we use to organize our sexual practices, identities and preferences, and the conventions for speaking and writing about them. How elaborately we are able to conceptualize a concept, and how effectively we can convey our sense of it to others, will depend on how rich or complex our language is.

Complexities of classification vary with historical and cultural context. The Kama Sutra, for example, has many words for sexual position, and the loss of this diversity is often attributed to colonization by the British, caricatured by their monolithic 'missionary position'. The ancient Greeks had words for different kinds of love, from sexual love to companionable love, but did not make the present-day distinction between homosexuality and heterosexuality. Nor did the Romans; sexual categories in ancient Rome were based on a distinction between active and passive. The penetrator was described as active, and the person penetrated was described as passive, with no reference to whether they were of the same or opposite sex.

Different vocabularies, different discourses

A range of different vocabularies is used to describe sexual behaviour, roughly divisible in most socio-cultural settings into more and less formal terms. Although boundaries are far from clear or fixed, we can distinguish technical terms (scientific and medical) from colloquial or vernacular language (which include euphemistic, slang, and taboo terms). Some examples are provided in Table 11.1. Sexuality is fairly unique in this respect. Using the analogy of eating again, the word 'eat' is in broad and acceptable currency – as likely to be read in medical journals as heard in a café.

Scientific discourses

Scientific or technical terms, often of Greek or Latin derivation, characterize expert discourses on sex. Many that are still in circulation today, such as *sado-masochism*, *paedophilia*, and *auto-eroticism*, were established by the early sexologists in the nineteenth

Table 11.1 Vocabularies used to describe sexual behaviour

Type of vocabulary	Examples of terms used
Formal	
Scientific	Copulate, coitus, heterosexual
Informal	
Colloquial	Have sex, to have/take (someone)
Euphemistic	Sleep with, go to bed with
Slang/obscene	Snog, shag, fuck

century – possibly in a quest to make the study of sexuality appear scientific. In general, they were interested in producing typologies of sexual perversions (Chapter 1). These included homosexuality and – a surprise to us now perhaps – heterosexuality. When this term was coined in 1869, it signified having sex with someone of the opposite sex for pleasure instead of procreation, which was seen as deviant. In the mid to late twentieth century, sexuality became a subject for broader scientific enquiry, in fields such as demography, medicine, psychology, and psychiatry, and a further tranche of scientific words entered the sexual lexicon, including *coitarche* and *coitus*, *menarche* and *menstruation*.

Indirect vocabularies

While the social patterning of sexual communication may be culturally specific, some universal features are discernible. In the English-speaking world, and in many former British colonies, verbal communication about sex is mostly indirect. Indirect speech commonly takes the form of euphemisms, with 'going to bed with' or 'sleep with' perhaps the best-known examples. Many basic verbs in the English language can take on sexual connotations in the appropriate context: the words 'have', 'come', 'give', 'take', 'make', and 'know' (as in the Biblical sense), for example.

Helen Lambert and Kate Wood used their research in India and South Africa respectively to compare modes of communication in different settings (Lambert and Wood, 2005). In Hindi-speaking regions of northern India, they note, sexual intercourse is referred to as 'meeting' (*milna*), 'sitting' (*baithna*) or, most commonly in reference to sex between married partners, 'conversing' (*bacit karna*) or 'speaking' (*bat karna*), while in the Xhosa-speaking context of South Africa's Eastern Cape, equivalent terms for sex include 'meeting', 'sleeping with', 'lying with', and words relating to loving. In relation to HIV, which is greatly feared, indirect communication is also codified in local expressions such as *amagama amathathu/amaw* ('the three/four letter thing'). Thus sexual expression is disguised in common, non-specific words, whose sexual meaning is only obvious in context. The use of terms whose meaning is ambiguous can be seen as yet another form of linguistic avoidance.

Experts indulge in their own form of indirect speech. Public health agencies, particularly at government level, tend to use what Lambert and Wood term 'dissociating' language. Typical words used in public discourse tend to be more formal, for example, 'penile-vaginal intercourse', 'oral-genital sex', and 'heterosexual activity'. Typical vocabularies include such terms as 'high risk', 'safer sex', and a proliferation of acronyms such as STI, MSM, and CSW. These terms may be difficult to map onto local terms and understandings.

Slang terms

Slang terms also proliferate in sexual expression. One way of distinguishing slang is that it is less often used in written or formal speech. The word 'fuck', for example, possibly the most ubiquitous slang term for sexual intercourse, has survived for centuries despite repression, since for large swathes of English history it would not have been seen in print (for a long time, the Oxford Etymological Dictionary completely ignored it). Many words that are considered slang today are early English words, which would once have been inoffensive, but which have come to be seen as terms of abuse.

The humour of slang, especially in sexual matters, helps to neutralize sensitive terms. This is seen in Cockney rhyming slang, where the sound of a similar-sounding inoffensive word replaces one that is less socially acceptable. Calling someone a 'berk' or 'burk' seems a relatively mild insult, but the term is in fact short for Berkshire, as in Berkshire Hunt, and is none other than rhyming slang (Richter, 1987).

Activity 11.2

Reflect on your reaction to seeing the words used in this text. Think about which words you feel comfortable using in different contexts. Why do you feel comfortable with some words and not others?

Feedback

In thinking about this, it is likely that you had different audiences or listeners in mind. How comfortable you felt with particular terms may well have been influenced by whether you had in mind a partner, colleagues, members of your family or friends. The next section explores this in greater detail.

Discourse as silence and repression

The vocabularies described above are very different, but all – the technical and the scientific, the euphemistic and the slang lexicons – in different ways can be seen to further the end of concealing what is being spoken about. Whether this is effected through making the term incomprehensible to the non-expert, as in the case of some technical terms, or by virtue of it not appearing in print or only being expressed in certain contexts, as in the case of swear words, or being so imprecise as to be concealed in conversation as in the case of euphemisms, the use of different vocabularies maintains the 'silence' that the philosopher Michel Foucault speaks of in relation to repression:

> We must try to determine the different ways of not saying such a thing ... There is not one but many silences, and they are an integral part of the strategies that underlie and permeate discourses.
>
> (Foucault, 1990: 27)

Foucault adds an extra layer of complexity to the simple distinction between what can and cannot be said. He urges us to examine the different ways of 'not saying things', who is allowed to use them and to whom. According to Foucault, the number of such discourses has proliferated over time:

> ...an immense verbosity is what our civilisation has required and organised. Surely no other type of society has ever accumulated – and in such a relatively short span of time – a similar quantity of discourses concerned with sex. It may well be that we talk about sex more than anything else.
>
> (Foucault, 1990: 33)

The reference to 'our civilisation' and a 'relatively short span of time' here should not be taken to mean that Foucault's 'veritable discursive explosion' has happened since Victorian times. On the contrary, he takes issue with such a view, dating the proliferation of discourses to the eighteenth century, and pointing out that societies and institutions representing extremes of sexual repression needed to produce copious amounts of discourse about sex for exactly that reason, since it was through discourse that legal and religious authorities defined which sexual behaviours were forbidden and which were permitted. The shift in the late eighteenth and nineteenth centuries in the West, from treating the regulation of sex as the exclusive concern of religious and legal authorities to treating it more properly as the concern of medical and scientific authorities, created yet more discourses.

Communication issues in context

In this section, we draw on some of our own research, and that of others, to illustrate and amplify some of the potential communication pitfalls of which practitioners need to be wary in three contexts:

1 Mounting a sexual health promotion intervention
2 Carrying out a sexual health consultation in clinical practice
3 Conducting sexual behaviour research.

Activity 11.3

As you read through each of the three contexts, consider the issues raised to date, think about their application in each case, and jot down some of the pitfalls sexual health practitioners need to be wary of in each.

Feedback

Compare your reflections with the points made below and make amendments or additions where necessary.

1. Mounting a sexual health promotion intervention

Commonly used sexual health messages, such as 'Just say no', 'Negotiate condom use', 'Discuss safer sex', 'Avoid penetrative sex', and 'Ask about your partner's sexual history', all assume a degree of communicational facility. A reluctance to talk explicitly about sex, both in interpersonal contexts and in official public health discourse, is the single most frequently cited social obstacle to sexual health promotion. Emphasis has often been placed on efforts to encourage communication (Gupta et al., 1996; Pliskin, 1997), yet Lambert and Wood (2005) caution against seeing this as an instant remedy. Calls for the promotion of communication skills and assertiveness, they say, may seem glib in settings in which social mores constrain communication about sex. In simply urging young people to talk about things, we may fail to recognize the powerful social norms constraining conversation. It is considered inappropriate for Xhosa parents in South Africa, and for Rajasthani parents in India, for example, to talk explicitly to one another about sex or other matters relating to reproduction (Lambert and Wood, 2005).

Strategies for the delivery of health promotional messages need to take account of not only the broader cultural settings in which sexual encounters occur, but the intimate dyadic context of sexual encounters. Health promotional advice of the 'Just say no' variety is particularly difficult to follow since, as conversation analysts remind us, accepting an invitation is interactionally more straightforward than declining one (Kitzinger and Frith, 1999). With regard to safer sex and condom use, the adoption of direct tactics is often urged, laying down rules clearly and unambiguously at the beginning of a sexual encounter.

Yet such a strategy may be at variance with personal goals, as evidenced by work carried out by Mitchell and Wellings (2002), in which young people were interviewed and asked to describe various aspects of their early sexual experience. The young people interviewed were often uncertain about their feelings for the other person, and about that person's feelings for them. They were also unsure about how far they would like to progress physically. A degree of communicational ambiguity served to safeguard self-esteem, protect against the possibility of rejection and the risk of making false assumptions, and allowed them to keep their options open. Thus there was some resistance to stating intentions clearly and definitively and this posed problems for the open discussion of sex. This is clearly incompatible with the discussion of safer sex practices, since talking about condoms is perceived as tantamount to assuming sex will occur. From the point at which condoms are mentioned for the first time, for example, there are clearly few opportunities for prevarication about whether or not to have sex. Mentioning a condom is often taken to indicate that sex is inevitable:

> Interviewer: What's wrong with just producing a condom?
> Respondent: You're just assuming that you'll have sex with someone, and you
> don't know whether they want to have sex with you.
>   (Young man aged 25–29 years)

2. Carrying out a sexual health consultation in clinical practice

Issues relating to language and terminology are apparent even before a sexual health service is approached. There are clear parallels between the euphemisms used in common parlance and the clinical nomenclature used to describe services. This was especially so in the past, in euphemistic terms such as 'special' clinic. In many countries today, the sexual health specialty is disguised as 'dermatology'. In others, the term sexually transmitted disease (STD) clinic has gradually been replaced by the term genito-urinary medicine (GUM) clinic, shifting the focus from the disease entity to a more neutral anatomical area, but one whose meaning, nevertheless, remains relatively inaccessible to users. The label 'family planning clinic' sends a cogent message that the prime purpose of contraception is to plan, space, and limit families, and this may deter young people merely aiming to avoid pregnancy. By the same token, there has been opposition to the term 'birth control' clinic, because of eugenic connotations.

There is evidence that in general clinical practice, sexual matters are spoken about less often than many young people would like. To address this, a research project was funded by the Medical Research Council to develop and pilot a tool aimed at improving sexual health communication in primary care (MacDowall et al., 2010). Focus group interviews were carried out with healthcare professionals in general practice to inform its design. The findings revealed high awareness among healthcare practitioners of the challenges of using appropriate and intelligible language.

Practitioner 1:   You are not going to start talking about sexual intercourse to a 14-year-old. You just say 'sex'.
Interviewer: Right.
Practitioner 2:   For some patients you use two words together … You say the proper word and then another word that they might understand, but in the same sentence to try to help them understand.
    (General practice in South West England)

Healthcare practitioners described their own struggles to understand the current sexual idiom and, conversely, the efforts made by young people to use medical terminology:

Practitioner 1:   At the high school, they come out with words, [you think] 'if you could say that again'. I've never heard it called that before in my life.
Practitioner 2:   It's difficult isn't it. A lot of them are saying vagina and things like that …
Practitioner 3:   They think, he's a doctor, I'm going to use proper words and they try very hard to use medical words. [Laughter]
    (General practice in South West England)

The researchers also probed the consequences of using different vocabularies:

Practitioner 1:   What would happen if you used the language that they might use to their friends, in the surgery – what would the reception be?
Practitioner 2:   I would be concerned that they'd think I was trying to be youthful. Or I was being too familiar or just too … sexual.
    (General practice in North England)

Note the practitioners' concerns about using the frank terminology of their young patients. Most of us feel free to candidly discuss our sexual experiences with only a small number of people whom we most likely consider intimate friends. Thus when a researcher, clinician or sex educator talks about personal experiences, they may, in so doing, be seen to be closing the social distance between professional and client/patient and as being inappropriately intimate. As Foucault pointed out: 'If sex is repressed … then the mere fact that one is speaking about it has the appearance of a deliberate transgression' (Foucault, 1990: 6). Slang terms for sexual behaviours and body parts are often considered offensive and generally inappropriate to the purpose, as are the more esoteric, formal terms.

3. Conducting sexual behaviour research

Many researchers, including Alfred Kinsey, have cautioned against the use of a standardized questionnaire and neutral terminology, advising instead the use of the vernacular terms used by participants.

> In order to have questions mean the same thing to different people, they must be modified to fit the vocabulary, the educational background, and the comprehension of each subject. It is especially important to use a vocabulary with which the subject will feel at home, and which he [sic] will understand.
>
> (Kinsey et al., 1948: 52)

Although this strategy has advantages in terms of achieving validity (see Chapter 15), researchers carrying out research into sexual behaviour 50 years later, with random probability rather than volunteer samples, decided to test these assumptions empirically. The team carrying out the British National Survey of Sexual Attitudes and Lifestyles carried out 50 in-depth interviews with men and women, exploring their preferences for the form and phrasing of questions. They found that understanding of technical terms was, indeed, partial:

Interviewer:	What about vaginal sex, do you know what that means?
Respondent:	No.
Interviewer:	And, penetrative sex?
Respondent:	No, haven't heard of it, um, is it sort of going half way?

(Single woman aged 19 years)

Respondent:	No, I don't know what that means.

(Married woman aged 46–55 years)

Respondent:	No, never heard of that actually.

(Single woman aged 25 years)

The problem was not simply one of understanding. Scientifically or medically arcane language was often thought to denote some kind of bizarre or unorthodox activity (Spencer et al., 1988) – not surprisingly perhaps, given the early link between these terms and perversion.

Interviewer:	Penetrative sex?
Respondent:	Well, I suppose it's something queers do is penetrating – penetrative sex.

(Married man aged 35 years)

> *Interviewer:*   Heterosexual?
>
> *Respondent:*   Well, it's all the same to me. Heterosexual, bisexual, they're all bloody queers as far as I'm concerned.
>
> (Single man aged 26–35 years)

What was classified as 'normal' sex was not seen as needing a distinguishing term to define it. At the same time, there was an aversion to the use of 'street' terms:

> *Interviewer:*   Should colloquial language be used?
>
> *Respondent:*   No, you've got to be very careful because if you try to come down to somebody's level too much … well, you've got to be very, very careful …
>
> (Single man aged 21–25 years)

The use of terms often varied within the account given by any one respondent, and the different terms used often signified qualitatively different experiences:

> You use different words as you go through life. Originally, you'll be – you know – 'get her knickers off' sort of thing, 'get her pants down' and then it probably goes on to 'I've had sex with her', 'I've screwed her' and later on when you've got a more permanent kind of relationship you might talk about 'making love'.
>
> (Married man aged 30–35 years)

To summarize, the researchers found that people do not always understand, and/or are unfamiliar with, technical sexual terminology; can be offended by 'street' terms used in 'inappropriate' contexts; may see scientific terms as referring to more bizarre or unorthodox practices; and use a variety of expressions according to who they are talking to and what is being described.

Indirect terms do not serve sexual health practitioners well, whether they are engaged in health promotion, clinical practice or research. They are too imprecise. In the wake of the then US president Bill Clinton's public denial that he had 'had sex' with White House intern Monica Lewinsky because no penile-vaginal intercourse had taken place, for example, researchers at the Kinsey Institute re-analysed the data they had collected in 1991 on the sexual lives of college students. The students had been asked 'Would you say you had sex with someone if the most intimate behaviour that you engaged in was x/y/z'. The results showed that when the most intimate behaviour engaged in was oral-genital sex contact, the response from two-thirds of students was 'No'. Thus if the term 'sex' was used in research, the majority of respondents would not include occasions of oral-genital sex.

Implications for sexual health practice

1 Attention needs to be paid to the fact that messages can be conveyed by silence and/or invisibility. What is not shown or spoken about will be striking by its absence. For example, using a banana or other object to demonstrate correct condom use states clearly that a more realistic representation of an erect penis is not allowed, a message that may be more powerful than the message to use a condom.

2 Interventions may inadvertently offend against local social mores by assuming that silence should be replaced with speech and may therefore meet with limited success.

3 Since most people are not used to speaking openly about sex, permission may need to be given and examples set by sexual health practitioners and researchers.

4 Terminology should be chosen to safeguard rapport between practitioner/ researcher and client/participant, and which both feel comfortable with. Slang terms for sexual behaviours and body parts are often considered offensive and unacceptable, while technical terms may be misunderstood or misinterpreted.

5 Qualitative research is needed to explore the meanings of particular terms for respondents, and standardized questionnaires used in quantitative research need to provide explicit operational definitions of the terms used.

6 Advice messages conveyed to young people need to be compatible with the reality of their relationships. Safer sex advice needs to take account of features of sexual communication (e.g. ambivalence/ambiguity) that may be incompatible with direct and explicit expression.

7 Use of everyday language may be less exclusionary and more effective than that which uses the biomedical language of international and national health agencies, which may have no local referents.

Summary

The fact that sexual behaviour is subject to more social rules and controls than most other behaviours has implications for communication. Communication about sexual matters is not easy in any social context, and in some it is especially difficult. Problems arise where different terms are used in different contexts to describe sexual phenomena, where speaking of some behaviours is socially disapproved or forbidden, and where words may be used to conceal meanings. Assumptions cannot be made, therefore, that advice on safer sex will be easily followed, that practitioners and patients will share a common language with which to discuss sexual matters, or that research will be carried out with communicational ease. Thought needs to be given to the challenges for sexual health investigation and intervention.

References

Foucault M (1979) The History of Sexuality: An Introduction. London: Allen Lane.

Gupta GR, Weiss E and Mane P (1996) Talking about sex: a prerequisite for AIDS prevention, in LD Long and EM Ankrah (eds.) Women's Experiences with HIV/AIDS: An International Perspective. New York: Columbia University Press.

Kinsey AA, Pomeroy W and Martin C (1948) Sexual Behavior in the Human Male. Philadelphia, PA: WB Saunders.

Kitzinger C and Frith HJ (1999) Just say no? The use of conversation analysis in developing a feminist perspective on sexual refusal, Discourse and Society, 10(3): 293–316.

Lambert H and Wood K (2005) A comparative analysis of communication about sex, health and sexual health in India and South Africa: implications for HIV prevention, Culture, Health and Sexuality, 7(6): 527–41.

MacDowall W, Parker R, Nanchahal K, Ford C, Lowbury R, Robinson A et al. (2010) 'Talking of sex': developing and piloting a sexual health communication tool for use in primary care, Patient Education and Counselling, 81(3): 332–7.

Mitchell K and Wellings K (2002) The role of ambiguity in sexual encounters between young people in England, Culture, Health and Sexuality, 4(4): 393–408.

Pliskin KL (1997) Verbal intercourse and sexual communication: impediments to STD prevention, *Medical Anthropology Quarterly*, 11(1): 89–109.

Richter A (1987) *The Language of Sexuality*. Jefferson, NC: McFarland.

Spencer L, Faulkner A and Keegan J (1988) *Talking About Sex*. London: SCPR.

Further reading

Cameron D and Kulick D (2003) *Language and Sexuality*. Cambridge: Cambridge University Press.

Promotion of sexual health

Martine Collumbien and Wendy MacDowall

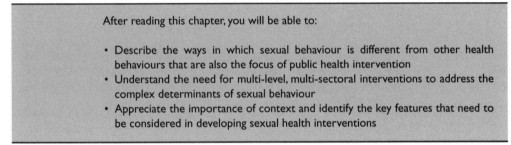

Overview

The aim of health promotion is to prevent illness and to promote health and wellbeing by encouraging healthy behaviours and by enabling individuals and communities to control wider environmental factors that determine their health. In this chapter, we discuss behaviour change as well as approaches to influencing social structures and barriers that constrain individual change. We start by considering the main approaches used in public health and we review communication strategies. We argue for implementing interventions at different levels and in different sectors. Showing the critical importance of context, we end by describing how to plan comprehensive sexual health promotion interventions.

Learning outcomes

After reading this chapter, you will be able to:

- Describe the ways in which sexual behaviour is different from other health behaviours that are also the focus of public health intervention
- Understand the need for multi-level, multi-sectoral interventions to address the complex determinants of sexual behaviour
- Appreciate the importance of context and identify the key features that need to be considered in developing sexual health interventions

Key terms

Behavioural intervention: Action(s) that aim to change behaviour by motivating, empowering, and/or persuading individuals, or groups of individuals, to adopt the desired behaviour(s).

Combination prevention: Combines behavioural, biomedical, and structural interventions to address the immediate risks and underlying causes of vulnerability to adverse sexual health outcomes.

Harm reduction: An approach that seeks to minimize avoidable harms associated with risky sexual behaviour. Harm reduction contrasts with approaches that seek to eradicate the behaviour.

Structural approaches Action(s) that aim to change the broader context that influences risk behaviour and vulnerability, by altering social, political, economic, and/or environmental factors.

Introduction

From a public health perspective, the goal of sexual health promotion is to improve the sexual health status of the population via social interventions. For those engaged in this endeavour, there are two fundamental questions: First, *what* specifically do we want to improve? And second, *how* are we going to do that? These seemingly simple questions belie the many challenges and complexities of modifying sexual behaviour. Some of these challenges and complexities are in fact common to all efforts to modify health-related behaviour but others are unique to sexual behaviour.

Activity 12.1

Based on your reading of the previous chapters:

- In what ways does sexual behaviour differ from other health behaviours, such as taking regular exercise and eating a balanced diet?
- How might each of these differences impact on attempts to modify sexual behaviour?

Feedback

Some of the key differences and their potential impacts include:

1 In all societies constraints are imposed on sexual behaviour, either via the law or socially. These may drive illegal or stigmatized behaviours underground, limit the extent to which people can act to protect their health, and/or limit service provision and prevention efforts.
2 Sexual health is a particularly sensitive topic for governments. These sensitivities influence the prioritization, and consequently the funding, of some issues and not others. Political positions can also influence the nature of the activities that are supported (such as the focus on abstinence under George Bush's Administration in the United States).
3 Communication about sexual behaviour presents many challenges for both the lay person and health professional alike, which can impede sexual health promotion in many different ways (see Chapter 11).
4 Sex takes place in private between the people involved, which makes it more difficult to regulate sexual behaviour by 'law'. Social stigmatization may keep unsafe or coercive behaviour from public view and from prevention efforts.

As you have learned in previous chapters, 'sexual health' is a broad term that encompasses a number of the major public health challenges the world faces. The World Health Organization (WHO, 2010) identifies the key elements as:

- sexually transmitted infections (STIs) including HIV, reproductive tract infections;
- unintended pregnancy and safe abortion;
- sexual dysfunctions and infertility;
- violence related to gender and sexuality (including female genital mutilation);

- young people's sexual health and sexual health education;
- sexual orientation and gender identity;
- mental health issues related to sexual health;
- the impact of physical disabilities and chronic illnesses on sexual wellbeing; and
- the promotion of safe and satisfying sexual experiences.

Many of these elements have whole chapters dedicated to them in this book and are not covered here. The points to note in relation to this chapter on interventions to promote sexual health are that (a) this is a daunting agenda and prioritization of efforts and resources will, and does, take place and (b) prioritization is not just driven by epidemiological imperatives; as noted above, political and cultural sensitivities will, and do, influence the process.

Activity 12.2

Taking the key elements of sexual health as defined by WHO (2010) listed above as your guide, think about the situation in your country:

- Which elements have received the most attention in terms of public health effort and which the least? Has there been any change in focus?
- Why do you think that is the case?

Feedback

It is likely that the adverse outcomes of sexual behaviour (STIs, HIV, and unintended pregnancy) have received the most attention in your country; indeed, they may be the sole focus. Sexual violence (Chapter 4) and sexual dysfunction (Chapter 5) are increasingly being addressed but 'shifting programmes from an exclusive focus on prevention, treatment and care of sexual ill-health to encompass broader concepts of health and well-being remains a challenge' (WHO, 2010: 19). Local cultural and sexual norms limit the extent to which sexually satisfying lifestyles can be promoted, as this goal requires explicit discussion of sexuality and its role in intimacy and well-being. But there are opportunities for raising issues of sexual satisfaction in treatment and care settings: people living with HIV, for instance, can be counselled to prevent harm to their partners by discussing sex more openly in order to make sex safer and satisfying. Explicit discussion of pleasure is more common in campaigns targeted at gay men in the West (Chapter 7), but generally avoided elsewhere. However, the progress in getting sexual rights on the public health agenda may affect what is feasible in future.

Approaches in public health

Generally, a liberal behavioural approach, focusing on harm limitation and relying on persuasion and social learning is favoured. However, responses calling for abstinence from sex, abolition of sex work, and punitive measures against those engaging in 'deviant' behaviour are prevalent, despite evidence that these may not benefit public health.

In sex work, the empowerment approach for sex workers (see the example of Sonagachi in Chapter 8) is most in line with principles of harm reduction. It respects sex work as a profession and helps women understand their human rights and legal entitlements. Such programmes are effective when they are sufficiently holistic and responsive to sex workers' needs. However, like any approach there is a disadvantage: they often fail to protect young women who may have been coerced or trafficked into sex work (Tucker and Tuminez, 2011).

The alternative strategy is abolitionism. Interventions using this approach prioritize criminalization over harm limitation. Many anti-trafficking campaigners support this and often conflate trafficking with sex work. This can lead to concerns about an influx of trafficked women during large-scale events like the Olympic Games. Despite the lack of evidence for this, police crackdowns lead to displacement of sex workers who then become more difficult to reach (Deering et al., 2012).

Rights-based approaches stress the need to curb abuses against stigmatized groups. Both UNAIDS and WHO strongly advocate them being at the core of prevention (WHO, 2010).

Behavioural interventions

Shifts in health communication have been towards multi-component, multi-level programmes (MacDowall and Mitchell, 2006). Such strategies are premised on the need to address the broader determinants of health (such as gender inequalities) that are often beyond individual control (MacDowall and Mitchell, 2006). Family Health International (FHI) used the term 'strategic behavioural communication' to describe this strategy (FHI, 2005). Specific interventions associated with this approach include peer education, counselling, support groups, mass media, traditional media, community mobilization, and advocacy. Individual health behaviour is not the only focus; strategies seek to influence the environment and delivering consistent messages to all stakeholders requires communication expertise.

Key communication approaches include the following:

- *Advocacy* includes changing public opinion by getting people in authority to speak up; by drawing attention to important issues; by promoting new policies in order to influence decision-makers in changing public policy; and by redefining norms. Chapter 10 emphasizes the need for a human rights approach to sexual health policy and practice.
- *Community mobilization* or community development is an important approach (or philosophy) in health promotion (Hargreaves and Twine, 2006) that seeks to empower communities to find solutions to their health needs. It involves facilitating collective action through a participatory process and is especially important for socially disadvantaged groups, including women, sex workers, gay men, and MSM.
- *The mass media* are used widely in HIV/AIDS prevention for promoting behaviour change, agenda setting, and shifting social norms. The main advantages are that it can reach a wide variety of people including hidden or hard-to-reach groups within the population. Mass media approaches can also raise public consciousness about health issues, bringing them to the attention of policy-makers and prompting public discussion. National coverage can help to legitimate additional strategies at local level, and may even trigger new initiatives. Although mass communication techniques are less suited to conveying complex information and to teaching skills, they can support other intervention components that are more effective at this.

Box 12.1 Using mass media to change social norms

Mass media can be particularly powerful in changing social norms and has been successfully used in stigma reduction campaigns. A soap opera in Botswana, 'The Bold and the Beautiful', with a 2-year HIV storyline, was credited with contributing to significant declines in levels of HIV stigma nationally (Mahajan et al., 2008). In South Africa, the television drama serial 'Soul City' used edutainment (in which messages about social issues are integrated into drama) to raise awareness of a range of HIV/AIDS-related issues. The series seeks to bring about change at the level of the individual (e.g. increasing knowledge), community (e.g. getting people to visit services), and society (e.g. influencing public policy). On domestic violence, 'Soul City' partnered social mobilization organizations to successfully advocate for the implementation of the Domestic Violence Act (Usdin et al., 2005). The success of edutainment is attributed to the fact that the audience can identify with the characters in the story. Modelling of positive norms and behaviours is also possible (Usdin et al., 2005).

Audiences do not consist of homogeneous groups and a single approach to risk reduction is unlikely to suit all. Individuals therefore need to be given a range of behavioural options to reduce their risk. For example, abstinence-only messages may be helpful to some young people, but abstinence is neither desired nor possible for others (such as those who are already married). Thus abstinence messages are best promoted alongside other messages about partner reduction and condom use.

Theory and context

Theories of communication and behaviour change are helpful in creating appropriate message strategies and in choosing the right vehicles in which to place messages. Derived mainly from behavioural sciences, these models highlight the importance of knowledge and beliefs about health, the importance of self-efficacy (the belief in one's competency to take action), and perceived social norms and social influences (as the individual places value on social approval or acceptance by different social groups). They also recognize that individuals in a population may be at different stages of change at any one time. The environment needs to be considered too – whether changing the environment or changing people's perception of the environment (Nutbeam and Harries, 2004). Interventions that use a theory-based approach are most effective (irrespective of the theory), mainly because they improve planning and delivery (Kelly, 2006).

The context, however, is critical and theoretical models underlying intervention in one setting may not translate to another. For example, models developed from empirical research in western settings and based on notions of individual autonomy have been shown to be less relevant in other cultures where individual identity is more grounded in family and community roles (Elder, 2001). Individual-level theories focusing on motivation and skills need to be integrated with theories that take account of the structural influences on behaviour (de Wit et al., 2011).

Ecological models view behaviour and environment as interacting in a reciprocal, 'cause-and-effect' way (FHI, 2005; Heise, 2011). They posit that no single factor 'causes' an adverse outcome; instead, outcomes result from many factors interacting at different levels. Which factors are most important depends on the local context.

Activity 12.3

Reflect on the factors that may cause a young girl to die from an unsafe abortion. What interventions could be put in place to reduce the prevalence of unsafe abortion?

Feedback

- *Factors that contributed to the woman having an unintended pregnancy in the first place:* strict norms against premarital sex may have led to her never receiving information on the risks of sex; contraceptives may be available to (or targeted at) married women only; she may have had no power to negotiate protection.
- *Factors that contributed to her undergoing an unsafe abortion:* to protect the honour of the family, she (or her relatives) may have decided to end the pregnancy, using a non-qualified provider so as to maintain secrecy; safe abortion care may not have been available or only available in public hospitals where providers are known to be judgemental and not respect confidentiality; once she was in a critical position, her family did not get her to hospital in time to save her life.
- *Interventions depend on the context, but would be needed across levels and sectors:* they may include advocacy to legalize abortion where it is illegal; making legal abortion services safer and training staff on confidentiality and non-stigmatizing attitudes; introducing medical abortion, which does not require invasive procedures; targeting young women with sex education awareness campaigns; setting up youth-friendly services; education and empowerment initiatives with girls.

Accepting that context is critical leads us naturally to the conclusion that strategies should seek to engender an environment that is as supportive as possible.

Structural approaches

In Chapter 10, we learned that the source of adverse outcomes in sexual health (and in public health more broadly) is often the social, political, and economic environments that shape the individual and community. Structural interventions thus 'promote health by altering the context in which health is produced and reproduced' (Blankenship et al., 2006: 59).

This implies a need for long-term interventions, and which go beyond public health to include broader social and economic development. Interventions need to address both proximate factors, which have a direct bearing on individual risk (such as migration), as well as more distant factors (such as the way a country is governed) (Gupta et al., 2008). Transformative approaches seek to change the context at a higher (distant) level by, for instance, changing social norms that prevent women negotiating safer sex. Enabling approaches seek to address proximate factors that prevent individuals from making desired behaviour changes, such as ensuring that sexual health services are acceptable and accessible. Table 12.1 shows examples of structural interventions at different levels of response and in different sectors.

Table 12.1 Examples of structural interventions by level and by sector

Level	Sector of intervention	Examples
National or regional (macro)	Legal/policy	Legalization of abortion services Decriminalization of HIV transmission and of homosexuality Legalization of sex work Legal protection against rape and gender-based violence Raise or enforce age at marriage 100% condom use policy
	Education	Provision of universal education
	Public health	Voluntary testing and counselling Provision of wider mix of contraception Improvement of coverage and provision of sexual health services
	Macro-economic	Economic development strategies (diversification of economy may reduce need for migration)
Community or group (meso)	Community development	Creating public spaces for young girls and/or boys Organizing women's groups Community mobilization of sex workers
	Socio-economic	Reducing school fees (to increase access to education)
	Socio-cultural	Group-based education focusing on gender roles and relationships
	Mass media	Stigma reduction messages using posters or television drama
Individual level (micro)	Education	Context-specific sex education messages
	Micro-economic	Conditional cash transfers Microfinance schemes

Source: Adapted from Parkhurst (2007).

Intended and unintended consequences: the case of economic empowerment

Structural interventions seem intuitively sensible, yet the evidence for their effectiveness has not always been consistent. They may also bring about unintended negative consequences or may have different effects in different contexts. An example is economic empowerment for women.

Activity 12.4

How would you argue that investing in women's economic empowerment can reduce the level of intimate partner violence? What might be the risks to this approach? You may wish to review Chapters 4 and 10 before completing this activity.

Feedback

It is plausible that as women gain access to jobs, they increase social and economic power and may be more able to leave violent partners (in the longer term). However, increased income for women may not necessarily translate into increased bargaining power. Indeed, when women start to challenge the power distribution in the household, violence may increase in the short term.

In fact, evidence for the effect of employment (or access to independent income) on women's risk of partner violence is inconsistent. This is because the effect partially depends on the relative economic position of the women's partner and how much the couple adhere to cultural expectations regarding women challenging the provider role. In Latin-American studies, violence increased only when women's income was higher than that of their husbands (Heise, 2011). A good understanding of the local context is required, as well as careful monitoring of how the population adapts to changes brought about by interventions.

Examples of economic empowerment strategies include microfinance and conditional cash transfers. Microfinance is a strategy based on group-based lending among women, providing small amounts of credit to start up small income-generating activities. The IMAGE study in South Africa, where poverty and gender inequalities critically challenge prevention efforts, integrated a 'Sisters in Life' curriculum into an existing microfinance initiative. The curriculum raises critical awareness about gender and HIV and promotes solidarity among women. A randomized controlled trial showed a 55% reduction in reported intimate partner violence, but no impact on HIV (Pronyk et al., 2006). There was some evidence that women's risk may have increased through increased social and sexual networking. The positive impact of IMAGE on empowerment and violence was more a function of the 'Sisters in Life' training programme than of the micro-credit component (Kim et al., 2009).

A range of cross-sectional studies in Bangladesh has shown negative effects of participation in micro-credit on domestic violence, especially in the short term (Heise, 2011). This was especially the case for those women who were among the first to gain employment, at a time when women's individual and collective empowerment had not yet become accepted at the community level (Koenig et al., 2003). This highlights the need to target not only individual women but also the community at large.

Summary

Sexual behaviour presents challenges for health promotion strategies because: it is politically sensitive; it is difficult to talk about; and it takes place in private. Public health professionals generally focus on harm limitation and rely on persuasion and social learning to minimize adverse outcomes. Theories of communication and behaviour change are helpful in creating effective strategies but need combining with ecological models that take better account of the interactions between individual and contextual factors. Because the source of adverse sexual health outcomes is often the social, political and economic environment, structural interventions are required that seek to alter the context in which behaviours take place. Structural interventions are often long-term and may be transformative (seeking to change distant factors such as norms) or enabling (seeking to address proximate factors such as health services). The context is often complex and interventions do not always work as anticipated. It is crucial therefore to look out for unintended consequences.

References

Blankenship KM, Friedman SR, Dworkin S and Mantelli E (2006) Structural interventions: concepts challenges and opportunities for research, *Journal of Urban Health*, 83(1): 59–72.

Deering KN, Chettiar J, Chan K, Taylor M, Montaner JSG and Shannon K (2012) Sex work and the public health impacts of the 2010 Olympic Games, *Sexually Transmitted Infections* (DOI: 10.1136/sextrans-2011-050235).

Elder JP (2001) Behavior Change & Public Health in the Developing World. Thousand Oaks, CA: Sage.

Family Health International (FHI) (2005) *Strategic Behavioural Communication (SBC) for HIV and AIDS: A Framework*. Arlington, VA: FHI.

Gupta GR, Parkhurst JO, Ogden JA, Aggleton P and Mahal A (2008) Structural approaches to HIV prevention, *Lancet*, 372(9640): 764–75.

Hargreaves JR and Twine R (2006) Community development, in W MacDowall, C Bonnell and M Davies (eds.) *Health Promotion Practice*. Maidenhead: Open University Press.

Heise L (2011) *What Works to Prevent Partner Violence? An Evidence Overview*. London: London School of Hygiene and Tropical Medicine. Available at: http://strive.lshtm.ac.uk/resources/what-works-prevent-partner-violence-evidence-overview.

Kelly MP (2006) Evidence-based health promotion, in M Davies and W MacDowall (eds.) *Health Promotion Theory*. Understanding Public Health Series. Maidenhead: Open University Press.

Kim J, Ferrari G, Abramsky T, Watts C, Hargreaves J, Morison L et al. (2009) Assessing the incremental effects of combining economic and health interventions: the IMAGE study in South Africa, *Bulletin of the World Health Organization*, 87: 824–32.

Koenig, M.A., et al., (2003) Women's status and domestic violence in rural Bangladesh: individual and community level effects, *Demography*, 40(2): 269–88.

MacDowall W and Mitchell K (2006) Sexual health communication: Letting young people have their say, in R Ingham and P Aggleton (eds.) *Contextualizing Young People's Sexuality: International Perspectives*. Abingdon: Routledge.

Mahajan AP, Sayles JN, Patel VA, Remien RH, Sawires SR, Ortiz DJ et al. (2008) Stigma in the HIV/AIDS epidemic: a review of the literature and recommendations for the way forward, *AIDS*, 22: S67–S79.

Nutbeam D and Harries E (2004) *Theory in a Nutshell*. Sydney, NSW: McGraw-Hill.

Parkhurst J (2007) *Analysis of Social Transformative/Structural Approaches to HIV Prevention*. London: London School of Hygiene and Tropical Medicine.

Pronyk P, Hargreaves JR, Kim JC, Morison LA, Phetla G, Watts C et al. (2006) Effect of a structural intervention for the prevention of intimate partner violence and HIV in rural South Africa: results of a cluster randomized trial, *Lancet*, 368: 1973–83.

Tucker JD and Tuminez AS (2011) Reframing the interpretation of sex worker health: a behavioral–structural approach, *Journal of Infectious Diseases*, 204(suppl. 5): S1206–10.

Usdin S, Scheepers E, Goldstein S and Japhet G (2005) Achieving social change on gender-based violence: a report on the impact evaluation of Soul City's fourth series, *Social Science and Medicine*, 61(11): 2434–45.

World Health Organization (WHO) (2010) *Developing Sexual Health Programmes: A Framework for Action*. Geneva: WHO.

13 Sex education: theory and practice

Simon Forrest and Kaye Wellings

Overview

In this chapter, we consider some of the theoretical and practical issues relating to the provision of sex education. We explore what sex education is and how social, political, and moral concerns influence its aims, design, and delivery. We discuss the features linked with the effectiveness of sex education in improving young people's sexual health and we consider some key issues in its provision. Finally, we examine the evidence for effectiveness of interventions and some of the challenges of demonstrating effectiveness.

Learning outcomes

After reading this chapter, you will be able to:

- Identify a range of influences on sex education
- Describe some of the challenges faced by policy-makers and practitioners in planning and implementing sex education
- Critically assess the evidence base for effectiveness of sex education in improving sexual health

Key term

School-based sex education: Structured interventions within educational settings that seek to equip young people with the knowledge and means to protect their sexual health.

Introduction

Sex education is the process by which people acquire information and ideas about sexuality, sexual health, and relationships. The process takes place over the whole life course and draws on a range of sources. These include family members, friends, sexual partners, health professionals, the mass media, literature, music, and jokes.

A public health approach to sex education is concerned with contributing to this process through provision of structured interventions whose purpose is to equip individuals with the means to protect and improve their sexual health. An important role for sex education is in correcting misinformation gleaned from other sources.

The term sex education is most commonly used to describe the process as it occurs within school. Focusing sex education on young people in school makes sense because young people are relatively easily reached in formal educational settings; they are excluded from many public health interventions aimed at adults; and they are also at a stage at which sexual attitudes and behaviours are not yet entrenched.

Personal communication aimed at improving sexual health can take place in a number of settings. Primary care professionals may provide information about sexual health in the course of a general health check, for example, and the media are a well-documented source of information about sexual matters to all ages. Since these channels are dealt with elsewhere in this book, the focus in this chapter is predominantly on school-based sex education.

What do we mean by sex education?

Although there is widespread recognition of the importance of educating young people about sexual matters, there is no single, universally agreed definition of sex education. The definition formulated by UNESCO includes reference to age appropriateness and social context:

> ...an age-appropriate, culturally relevant approach to teaching about sex and relationships by providing scientifically accurate, realistic, non-judgemental information. Sexuality education provides opportunities to explore one's own values and attitudes and to build decision-making, communication and risk reduction skills about many aspects of sexuality.
>
> (UNESCO, 2009: 2)

In Sweden, one of the earliest countries to introduce sex education, the Swedish Association for Sexuality Education (RFSU) offers the following formulation:

> Sexuality education should support and prepare young people for leading a responsible sexual life. It should enable each and every individual to work towards learning how he/she wants to live and towards discovering what is right or wrong for him/her. The objectives of sexuality education are several; for example preventing STIs, unwanted pregnancies, loosening up gender stereotypes ... and also working against discrimination of LGBT-people ... pupils should also learn to respect other people's opinions and choices regarding sexuality and form of social life.
>
> (Olson, 2010)

The British Government describes sex and relationships education as:

> ...life-long learning about physical, moral and emotional development. It is about the understanding of the importance of marriage for family life, stable and loving relationships, respect, love and care. It is also about the teaching of sex, sexuality and sexual health. It is not about the promotion of sexual orientation or sexual activity – this would be inappropriate teaching.
>
> (Department for Education and Employment, 2000)

Activity 13.1

How do the above definitions vary, and what do they reveal about the social and political concerns underlying them?

Feedback

The UNESCO definition adopts a relativistic stance, recognizing diversity and accepting that the approach adopted will not be the same in all contexts and that the right age for receipt of sex education will vary from one individual to another, and from one society to another. Emphasis is also placed on the importance of adopting a non-judgemental position and of building skills as well as conveying information. The tone is experiential rather than didactic.

The RFSU guidance is also non-judgemental, the emphasis being on individual choice and autonomy, but it stresses responsibility and underscores the importance of respect for others. This definition includes some biomedical endpoints, notably preventing sexually transmitted infections (STIs) and unintended pregnancy, but it also includes protecting against discrimination and promoting tolerance.

The Department for Education and Employment definition places greater emphasis on sex within relationships. It is the only definition to mention marriage. In the last sentence, in which it is stipulated that sexual orientation or activity should not be promoted, we get a sense of concern to reassure those who might otherwise see sex education as encouraging diversity and experimentation and undermining traditional values.

Ideological perspectives are also apparent in the terms used for sex education. The term 'family life education', for example, commonly used in Eastern European countries that include Slovakia, Poland, and Hungary, implies that sex education is preparing young people for married life with children. The choice of name may be strategic, taking account of what impression is likely to lead to least resistance in a specific context (Parker and Wellings, 2006). Changes in labelling also reveal shifts in priorities over time. With the advent of the HIV/AIDS epidemic, for example, and recognition of the importance of sex education in preventing HIV transmission, names of sex education programmes were often changed to include the term 'health education'.

A controversial area of the curriculum

One reason for there being no single shared vision for sex education is that it is not a value-free activity, but one that has to take account of prevailing ideas about sexual identities and lifestyles in specific settings. In very few, if any, social contexts has sex education been free from controversy. Many of the issues currently critical in debates about sex education – whether or not it encourages 'precocious' sexual experimentation, who should be responsible for its teaching, and at what age it should start – have long exercised the minds of educators. More than a century ago, Freud, asked for his opinion on sex education, replied:

...what can be the purpose of withholding from children ... enlightenment ... about the sexual life of human beings? Is it from fear of arousing their interest in these matters prematurely, before it awakens in them spontaneously? Is it from a hope that concealment of this kind may retard the sexual instinct altogether until such time as it can find its way into the channels open to it in our middle-class social order? ... Is it possible that the knowledge which is withheld from them will not reach them in other ways? Or is it genuinely and seriously intended that later on they should regard everything to do with sex as something degraded and detestable from which their parents and teacher wished to keep them away as long as possible?

(Freud, 1907: 173)

At the time Freud was writing, at the turn of the twentieth century, sexual desire was seen as a potentially dangerous force from which young people needed protection (Chapter 1). Consequently, the focus of a great deal of sex education material from the early modern period was on instilling sexual abstinence until marriage and channelling children's sexuality into stereotypical sex and social roles in preparation for lives as husband or wife, engaging in sex primarily as a reproductive activity (Sauerteig and Davidson, 2009).

Today, still, there are very few countries in which sex education is universally accepted. Even in countries such as the Netherlands and Sweden, where sex education has been more widely accepted, its teaching is opposed by some religions, such as the Muslim and Catholic faiths. Much has been achieved by actively involving religious organizations as partners in sex education programmes and by working to alter wider social norms through other public health-related activities.

Activity 13.2

Opposition to sex education may be expressed via sensationalist media coverage. A sample of headlines from two conservative-leaning British newspapers is shown below. Think about the language used. What messages are these headlines attempting to convey?

The Daily Mail
Sex education teacher admits to double life as porn star (12 July, 2010)
Parent's anger after class of seven-year-olds is shown 'graphic sex cartoon' at school (10 June, 2010)
Children 'to be given compulsory sex education from age four' (5 July 2008)

The Telegraph
Primary school pupils exposed to 'explicit' sex advice (9 March 2011)
Parents describe sex education video for primary schools as 'disturbing' (11 May 2010)

Feedback

The first headline seeks to evoke fear about the type of person who might be teaching sex education. Terms such as 'explicit', 'graphic', and 'disturbing' are usually used to describe sexual content that is unsuitable for children and are deliberately employed here to invoke fear. The term 'exposed' is used in the sense of being exposed to a risk; the risk being sex education. The term 'compulsory' suggests to parents the supposed lack of control they have regarding what and how their children are taught.

Framing sex education

Whether explicitly or implicitly, sex education programmes may be organized around and framed by several discourses.

Disease prevention

Concerns about the spread and effects of STIs have long been the rationale for sex education. In the late nineteenth and early twentieth centuries, when syphilis was thought to account for around 10% of all hospital admissions in New York, the American Society for Sanitary and Moral Prophylaxis argued for primary prevention through provision of school-based sex education, emphasizing the dangers of sex, discouraging sexual activity until marriage, and providing instruction about human anatomy and physiology. The emergence of HIV/AIDS in the 1980s again galvanized interest in, and support for, sex education. In 1986, the United States Surgeon General recommended specific attention be given to HIV/AIDS in school-based sex education programmes. The importance of sex education in this context has since been highlighted in a number of international recommendations and indicators identified to monitor progress towards tested goals. At the United Nations General Assembly Special Session (UNGASS) on HIV/AIDS in June 2001, it was reported that fewer than 40% of young people aged 15—24 years possessed comprehensive knowledge about sexual health matters (UNGASS indicator 13) (Coates et al., 2008).

Population control and social welfare

Sex education may be seen as an important component of government-led population control strategies. China's 'one-child' policy, for example, which has traditionally relied on provision of contraception and abortion, is increasingly supplemented by sex education to enhance knowledge about fertility control. In many industrialized countries, teenage pregnancy is a strong policy focus (see Chapter 3), and sex education may be advocated as a means of equipping young people with knowledge and skills to prevent early pregnancy. Sex education was a principal component of strategies to prevent teenage pregnancy in France and the UK at the start of the twenty-first century.

'Traditional' moral values

The inculcation of moral values in the sense of teaching respect for self and others, recognizing equality and diversity, and honouring people's right to privacy and autonomy, are ideally intrinsic to all sex education. But sex education that explicitly stresses 'traditional' moral values generally emphasizes the sanctity of sex within marriage, and is concerned to instil in young people a set of values and beliefs relating to love and marriage.

A rights-based agenda

Public health approaches often engage with rights-based arguments. Providing sex education is seen as observing young people's right to receive information on sexual matters and to enjoy their sexuality and relationships. Rights-based arguments may be used to lobby for sex education or for inclusion of specific topics within programmes. Sex education can sometimes challenge prevailing statutory or legal regulations around sexual behaviours and identities (e.g. laws relating to the age of sexual consent, sexual practices or identities), and sometimes contributes to changes in the legislative context. For instance, using sex education to support HIV prevention may involve recognition of young people's need to attend sexual health services despite being under the age of sexual consent.

What makes a successful sex education programme?

Ideally, sex education should take place as part of a broader public health response to the promotion of sexual health. This will involve seeking to engage not only with schools but other youth settings, together with families and community leaders, and linking to broader activities including use of the media and provision of sexual health services. There will be a need to build consensus around the public health response by consulting with a range of individuals and organizations, including teachers, parents, social and youth workers; representatives of cultural, ethnic and faith groups, and a range of media providers and health professionals.

Challenges to sex education

Sex education may be more or less problematic according to the setting in which it is carried out. Many of the challenges faced when implementing programmes are associated with the moral and cultural climate surrounding sexuality in any context, structural problems involved in delivery, and resources and capacity to implement programmes. The example of the Mema kwa Vijana programme in Tanzania (see Box 13.1) illustrates some of these challenges in a resource-poor setting.

Box 13.1 Mema kwa Vijana (MkV) sexual health programme, Tanzania

The project *Mema kwa Vijana* ('Good things for young people' in Kiswahili) was set up in the Mwanza region of north-west Tanzania by AMREF, an international African organization, to help young people protect their sexual health. HIV/AIDS is a serious problem in Tanzania, affecting 7% of adults and transmission rates are high among young people. The project ran from 2004 to 2007 and aimed to reach half a million school children aged 12–19 years, at school and in sexual health services in four districts. Training was provided to teachers, to staff from the Ministry of

Education, and to health workers to provide youth-friendly sexual health services, and awareness of adolescent health issues was raised at local government level.

The project as a whole was evaluated by means of a randomized controlled trial, complemented by the HALIRA study, which investigated the processes by which MkV components were delivered. The study exposed serious challenges in using primary schools as a means of reaching young people with sexual health messages. These included:

* Low school attendance rates among pupils, which compromised HIV and sex education.
* Limited teaching skills and resources, despite training.
* Behaviours on the part of teachers with the potential to alienate pupils and parents, such as alcohol or sexual abuse.
* Teachers' difficulties in adapting to less didactic teaching styles, despite expertise in relaying information.
* Limitations of peer educators as informal educators and as models of behaviour to be emulated.

(Plummer et al., 2007)

Commonly raised questions

Despite contextual differences, the key questions raised in implementing sex education interventions are common to most countries. These include how best to facilitate implementation and overcome opposition, in which area of the curriculum it is to be taught, at what age and by whom, and what should be the key messages.

When should sex education begin?

Research has shown it is easier to promote healthy sexual behaviours before their onset than after they are established. There is no evidence that early introduction hastens the onset of sexual activity (Somers and Eaves, 2002) as some fear, and an early start also provides opportunities for clear, consistent, and accurate messages to be conveyed before young people are exposed to other sources, including, increasingly, the Internet and – relatedly – pornography. Ideally, provision of sex education should be needs-driven, that is, it should be provided in response to questions as they are raised by young people. However, the organization of the curriculum into blocks, and individual differences in needs, can make this impractical.

Who should teach sex education?

The most common pattern is for school teachers themselves to provide sex education. Training has been shown to be essential to the success of sex education programmes, but not all teachers are adequately prepared to teach the subject and some feel uncomfortable doing so (Wight et al., 2002).

Peer-led sex education techniques offer an alternative to teacher-led approaches, but are not widely used. The evidence suggests that they are popular with young people, and may increase knowledge, but have only marginal benefits in terms of uptake of risk reduction practice (Stephenson et al., 2004; Huang et al., 2008).

Doctors, school nurses, and other health professionals are rarely involved in sex education, though the case has been made for their role in recognizing problems such as abuse and unplanned pregnancy. Similarly, pupil visits to health settings outside of school are not common, despite evidence that sex education is more effective when linked with local sexual health services (HDA, 2001). Voluntary organizations feature prominently among agencies brought into schools to teach sex education, and offer advantages in allowing statutory agencies to distance themselves from what may be seen as a sensitive area of the curriculum (Parker and Wellings, 2006).

In which area of the curriculum should sex education be taught?

Although many believe that the teaching of sex education should be cross-curricular, at all grades, in practice this is rare. Typically, sexuality education is taught in biology lessons, and often in one other area of the curriculum – religious studies – as citizenship or health education. The widespread pattern of timetabling sexuality education in biology lessons reflects a pervasive emphasis on health-related aspects of sex, and a weaker focus on the psychosocial aspects. The evidence is that this is the reverse of what young people themselves want (MacDowall et al., 2006). Research shows that they favour an approach that goes beyond a simple mechanistic coverage of the biological facts of sex and reproduction, and provides guidance on relationships and the social and emotional aspects of sex.

Sex education does not have to be scheduled within the school timetable. Research has shown extra-curricular engagement with young people at increased risk of sexual vulnerability and ill health to be more effective. One of only four interventions showing declines in teenage pregnancy attributable to sex education programmes assigned disadvantaged 13- to 15-year-olds in New York City to their usual youth programme or to a year-round after-school programme: CAS-Carrera, with a comprehensive youth development orientation (Philliber et al., 2002).

What messages should be conveyed?

One of the most hotly debated questions is what should be the dominant messages transmitted to young people. As discussed in Chapter 12, the ideal in sexual health promotion is to formulate a hierarchy of messages, tailored to different audiences. In the context of sex education, these could include advice not to have sex, to practise safer (i.e. non-penetrative) sex where sexual activity has already been initiated, and to use condoms and other methods of contraception where sexual intercourse is established.

In practice, only the first and last of these messages have proved feasible in the context of sex education. Despite evidence that the benefits to public health of non-penetrative sexual practices (such as mutual masturbation) may be as significant as those of condom use (Donovan and Ross, 2000), non-penetrative sex rarely features in sexual health messaging. Indeed, in the USA, the practice of non-penetrative sex among young people has been met with concern rather than support (Biddlecom, 2004; Anonymous, 2005), while in the UK, the rare attempts that have been made to introduce information about non-penetrative practices into sex education – such as the suggestion made by the originators of the APAUSE sex education programme to introduce the idea of 'outercourse' – have met with outrage or derision (Hartley, 2003).

Thus sex education programmes have tended to polarize into those focusing on risk avoidance on the one hand, and risk reduction (or harm limitation) on the other. Characteristic of the first category are abstinence-based sex education in which the dominant message to young people has been to refrain from sex. In the second category are comprehensive sex education programmes, in which the dominant messages relate to risk reduction such as contraception and condom use. The two are not always mutually exclusive. So-called 'abstinence-plus' sex education programmes include risk reduction messages, and many comprehensive sex education programmes stress the importance of readiness for sex.

In terms of general principles, an unconditional 'no' message can be seen to be less feasible in the case of sex than in other risk behaviours, such as alcohol, tobacco or drug use. Since sexual activity is essential to survival, abstinence messages must be phrased not in terms of whether to have sex but when, and as we have seen, this tends to be variously qualified in terms of marriage, age or readiness (Chapter 6).

Some studies have shown an association between abstinence-only sex education and delayed sexual initiation, but this is not confirmed by systematic reviews. Other studies (Brückner and Bearman, 2005) have shown that when young people given abstinence-only sex education did start to have sex, it was significantly less likely to be protected, supporting a systematic review in which four out of five sex education programmes found to have an adverse impact in terms of sexual health outcomes were abstinence-only (DiCenso et al., 2002).

Kirby et al. (2007) interpret the research on sex education to suggest that sex education programmes should:

- be guided by theories of social learning and health-related behaviour;
- provide basic, accurate information about the risks of unprotected intercourse and methods of avoiding unprotected intercourse;
- address social or media influences on sexual behaviours;
- provide practice in communication and negotiation skills;
- introduce sex education before patterns of sexual behaviour are established;
- adopt a sex-positive, as opposed to a sex-negative, tone;
- challenge discriminatory views and behaviour including sexism and homophobia;
- take account of young people's needs, including those relating to existing sex education and sexual health services.

Is school sex education effective?

Before considering the answer to this question, we should note that the question itself is not routinely asked in relation to other subjects in the school curriculum. Whether school leavers subsequently practise the foreign language they have learnt, or put into use the design and technology skills they have acquired, is not generally seen as a priority area for research. This may in part be because sex education is increasingly seen as a public health intervention, and thus requires evaluation, not least to assess cost-effectiveness. But it may also reflect political concerns forcing a demonstration of efficacy for a curriculum subject whose value is in question.

The crucial question is what goals need to be achieved for sex education to be deemed successful. The measurement of effectiveness will depend on the outcomes regarded as valid. Some see only hard, distal outcomes such as STIs and unplanned pregnancies as legitimate. Others accept achievement of the more proximate indicators (such as reductions in risk behaviours) or psychosocial endpoints (such as improvements in self-esteem, self-efficacy or sexual decision-making skills) as proof of success. However, even where the intended goals are proximate ones, there may still be pressure to demonstrate an impact on the downstream, biomedical goals.

One important – but often overlooked – psychosocial endpoint is the extent to which sex education programmes foster future 'physical, emotional, and social wellbeing in relation to sexuality' (WHO, 2006). Although the WHO definition of sexual health explicitly mentions pleasurable sexual experiences, the attainment of sexual wellbeing in this sense is generally ignored as a potentially valid endpoint for evaluation (Ingham, 2005). An explicit focus on pleasure is likely to be opposed in most cultures (Ingham, 2005). However, broader discussion about the meaning of positive sexual experience – touching on issues such as masturbation, acceptance of one's sexuality, feelings about one's body, and guilt and shame in relation to sex – may be justified as contributing to future sexual wellbeing (Ingham, 2005; see also Chapter 5).

There is often pressure, too, to show that sex education does not have unintended and undesirable outcomes. While some believe that provision enables young people to make informed choices and to protect their sexual health, others take the view that it hastens onset of sexual activity, increases risk-taking, and encourages early experimentation.

The public health benefit of sex education has, until recently, been unclear. The evidence base consisted largely of isolated studies of different design and their findings were inconclusive. Not surprisingly, perhaps, there are as many interpretations of the evidence as there are opinions held and, until recently, research has offered scope for different interpretations. Some studies have attributed to sex education a reduction in risk behaviours, some have shown no effect, and yet others have shown an increase. Thus advocates and opponents alike have been able to selectively dismiss empirical studies as flawed or embrace them as valid, according to whether or not they support their stance on the issue.

Publication of several systematic reviews of the effectiveness of sex education programmes at the start of the twentieth century put the evidence base on a more robust footing (DiCenso et al., 2002). Such reviews have shown school-based sex education to lead to improved awareness of risk and knowledge of risk reduction strategies. They also provide evidence that school-based sex education does not hasten onset of sexual behaviour or increase risk-taking as some have feared. Yet the demonstrable effects of school-based sex education on sexual ill health are modest. The reviews conclude that, overall, sex education interventions neither delay initiation of sexual intercourse, nor improve risk reduction practice or reduce pregnancy or STI rates in young people (DiCenso et al., 2002).

Activity 13.3

Might one reason for the apparent lack of impact result from the methods used to evaluate sex education programmes? Randomized controlled trials (RCTs) are increasingly seen as the gold standard evaluation technique. Yet the evidence for the effectiveness of sex education from systematic reviews of RCTs is disappointing. List some reasons why RCTs might not be ideally suited to assessing the effectiveness of sex education programmes.

Feedback

1. *Strength of effect/potency.* Sex education differs from clinical interventions involving, say, medication or surgery, in which exposed and control groups are easily distinguished. It is unusual to find a school in which no sex education of any kind is included in the curriculum, so that there is no truly unexposed population. What tends to be trialled is a *type* of sex education, perhaps peer-led, or conveying a particular message, and the comparison is with what is routinely provided. What is then being measured is the increment of effect that might accrue to receipt of a particular programme component, which is likely to be small.

2. *Power.* Outcomes chosen for measurement of effectiveness, such as STIs, may be too rare/relatively uncommon for studies to be powered to find an effect, given the limitations of cost on sample size.

3. *Feasibility.* Outcomes chosen for measurement of effectiveness, say teenage pregnancy, may be too far downstream for the evaluation research to capture them, given the time scale of the evaluation research.

4. *Sensitivity and attribution.* Sex education programmes stand more chance of success when they are part of multi-faceted interventions, which might include media campaigns and enhanced sexual health services. Where intervention components are population-wide, there will be no groups without exposure and, moreover, the interaction between the different programme components will make it difficult to single out the effects of sex education.

5. *Contamination.* Schools are not closed institutions; their pupils meet in pubs, clubs, and in friendship groups involving those from other schools. So sex education messages will not only reach those who hear them in school. The resulting contamination may be beneficial in terms of diffusion of health promotional messages, but will be problematic for the evaluation.

6. *Fidelity.* At the early stages of their development, many sex education programmes employ specially skilled and committed staff and these qualities may not be replicated in the broader range of practitioners once the programme is rolled out, leading potentially to problems of 'fidelity' in replicating the programme (see Chapter 16).

Evaluating the impact of sex education programmes is difficult. Ideally, evaluation research needs to have longer-term follow-up to help improve understanding of effects on longer-term outcomes, and thorough process evaluation to monitor implementation and assess reception by young people. Evaluations may need to move away from the pursuit of narrow, biomedical outcomes linked causally to sex education, to find ways of assessing and reflecting the effects of wider social and environmental factors.

One unintended and undesirable effect of the increasing move towards RCTs to assess the impact of sex education is that programmes found to have little or no effect in trials, even if this is attributed to some of the factors mentioned above, tend not to be taken up, while those that have not been rigorously evaluated may well be rolled out. As we explain in Chapter 16, less rigorous evaluations are more likely to show positive results. Many sex education programmes are not subjected to critical, robust evaluation because resources for evaluation were not integrated into the planning and commissioning stages, and these are unlikely to be the best programmes.

Summary

Sex education is the lifelong process by which people learn about sexuality from a wide range of sources. Public health seeks to contribute to this process through structured interventions aimed at improving sexual health. Formal educational settings are able to target young people prior to them establishing sexual relationships and behaviours, and at a time when they are less easily targeted in other settings.

Sex education is not a value-free enterprise and programme content may be influenced by moral beliefs about what is right and wrong, by cultural attitudes to sexual identities and rights, and by government policies on the control of STIs and population control. Such influences need to be taken into account when designing programmes. Educational interventions need to be age appropriate, delivered by those most competent to do so, and ideally should take place across the curriculum and at all ages. The messages should be feasible and likely to help young people avoid risk.

Sex education should be seen not in isolation but as an important component in broader initiatives to improve the health and wellbeing of young people. Used in isolation, experimental methods of evaluating its effectiveness, such as RCTs, may not be adequate to assess impact and may need to be supplemented by methods better suited to the evaluation of complex interventions.

References

Anonymous (2005) Warning: teenagers may view non-coital sex as a safe option, *Contraceptive Technology Update*, 26(6): 4.

Biddlecom AE (2004) Trends in sexual behaviours and infections among young people in the United States, *Sexually Transmitted Infections*, 80(suppl. 2): ii74–ii79.

Brückner H and Bearman PS (2005) After the promise: the STD consequences of adolescent virginity pledges, *Journal of Adolescent Health*, 36: 271–8.

Coates TJ, Richter L and Caceres C (2008) Behavioural strategies to reduce HIV transmission: how to make them work better, *Lancet*, 372(9639): 669–84.

Department for Education and Employment (2000) *Sex and Relationships Education Guidance 7/2000*. London: DfEE.

DiCenso A, Guyatt G, Willan A and Griffith L (2002) Interventions to reduce unintended pregnancies among adolescents: systematic review of randomised controlled trials, *British Medical Journal*, 324: 1426–35.

Donovan B and Ross MW (2000) Preventing HIV: determinants of sexual behaviour, *Lancet*, 355(9218): 1897–901.

Freud S (1907) The sexual enlightenment of children (An open letter to Dr M. Furst), in *On Sexuality: Three Essays on the Theory of Sexuality and Other Works*. Pelican Freud Library Vol. 7. Harmondsworth: Penguin.

Hartley C (2003) Government backs oral sex lessons for the under-16s, *The Sun*, 21 February.

Health Development Agency (HDA) (2001) *Teenage Pregnancy: An Update on Key Characteristics of Effective Interventions*. London: HDA.

Huang H, Ye X, Cai Y, Shen L, Xu G, Shi R et al. (2008) Study on peer-led school-based HIV/AIDS prevention among youths in a medium-sized city in China, *International Journal of STD and AIDS*, 19(5): 342–6.

Ingham R (2005) 'We didn't cover that at school': education against pleasure or education for pleasure?, *Sex Education*, 5(4): 375–88.

Kirby D, Laris B and Rolleri L (2007) Sex and HIV education programs: their impact on sexual behaviors of young people throughout the world, *Journal of Adolescent Health*, 40: 206–17.

MacDowall W, Wellings K, Mercer CH, Nanchahal K, Copas AJ, McManus S et al. (2006) Learning about sex: Results from Natsal 2000, *Journal of Health Education and Behaviour*, 33: 802–11.

Olson H (2010) *Knowledge, Reflection and Dialogue: Swedish Sexuality Education in Brief.* Available at: http://www.rfsu.se/en/Engelska/Sexuality-Education/Knowledge-reflection-and-dialogue/ (accessed 21 April 2011).

Parker R and Wellings K (2006) *Sex Education in Europe: The SAFE Project.* Brussels: IPPF European Network.

Philliber S, Kaye JW, Herrling S and West E (2002) Preventing pregnancy and improving health care access among teenagers: an evaluation of the children's aid society-carrera program, *Perspectives on Sexual and Reproductive Health*, 34: 244–51.

Plummer M, Wight D, Wamoyi J, Nyalali K, Ingall K, Mshana G et al. (2007) Are schools a good setting for adolescent sexual health promotion in rural Africa? A qualitative assessment from Tanzania, *Health Education Research: Theory and Practice*, 22: 483–99.

Sauerteig LDH and Davidson R (eds.) (2009) *Shaping Sexual Knowledge: A Cultural History of Sex Education in Twentieth Century Europe.* London: Routledge.

Somers CL and Eaves MW (2002) Is earlier sex education harmful? An analysis of the timing of school-based sex education and adolescent sexual behaviours, *Research in Education*, 67: 23–32.

Stephenson JM, Strange V, Forrest S, Oakley A, Copas A, Allen E et al. (2004) Pupil-led sex education in England (RIPPLE study): cluster-randomised intervention trial, *Lancet*, 364(9431): 338–46.

UNESCO (2009) *International Technical Guidance on Sexuality Education: An Evidence-informed Approach for Schools, Teachers and Health Educators.* Section on HIV and AIDS, Division for the Coordination of UN Priorities in Education. Paris: UNESCO.

Wight D, Raab GM, Henderson M, Abraham C, Buston K, Hart G et al. (2002) Limits of teacher delivered sex education: interim behavioural outcomes from randomised trial, *British Medical Journal*, 324: 1430.

World Health Organization (WHO) (2006) *Defining Sexual Health.* Report of a Technical Consultation on Sexual Health, 28–31 January 2002. Geneva: WHO. Available at: http://www.who.int/reproductive-health/publications/sexualhealth/index.html (accessed 31 January 2012).

Further reading

Forrest S, Strange V, Oakley A and the RIPPLE Study Team (2002) A comparison of students' evaluations of a peer-delivered sex education programme and teacher-led programme, *Sex Education*, 2(3): 195–214.

Lindberg L, Santelli JS and Singh S (2006) Changes in formal sex education: 1995–2002, *Perspectives on Sexual and Reproductive Health*, 38: 182–9.

Milburn K (1995) A critical review of peer education with young people with special reference to sexual health, *Health Education Research*, 10(4): 407–20.

Ogden J and Harden A (1999) The timing, format and content of school-based sex education: an experience with a lasting effect?, *British Journal of Family Planning*, 25: 115–18.

Sexual health services

Rebecca French and Kirstin Mitchell

Overview

The provision of adequate and appropriate sexual health services plays a vital role in public health interventions aimed at improving sexual health. In this chapter, we examine their role and the different means of their delivery, including the merits of adopting a more integrated approach to sexual health care. We conclude by examining some of the barriers that prevent people accessing services, and explore interventions to overcome these barriers.

Learning outcomes

After reading this chapter, you will be able to:

- Describe the role of sexual health services
- Explain the principles of integration of sexual health services, and appraise the case for and against 'one-stop shops'
- Identify the key barriers to using sexual health services, and interventions to address these barriers

Key terms

One-stop shop: Sexual health services offering a comprehensive range of services under one roof, even though services may be provided by different health professionals or within different clinics.

Service users: A range of terms is used to describe users of sexual health services, including patients, consumers, and clients. Since people attend services for a variety of reasons, the term 'service user' is employed in this chapter.

The role of sexual health services

Sexual health services should be effective, convenient, of high quality, and accessible to all. Unfortunately, high rates of morbidity and mortality are still associated with inadequate and poor-quality sexual and reproductive health services in some areas of the world (WHO, 2010).

Ideally, sexual health services would be provided to ensure that all facets of sexual health are addressed (Chapter 1). In practice, services to treat and control sexually transmitted infections/HIV, to prevent unplanned pregnancy, and to provide safe abortion are more common than those to address sexual violence or to promote sexual health. Each of the main roles and responsibilities is described below.

Prevention, control, and treatment of sexually transmitted infection and HIV

Sexual health services should include prompt and effective management of sexually transmitted infections (STIs) and HIV (Medfash, 2005; WHO, 2007) as well as reproductive tract infections (RTIs).

The effective diagnosis of STIs requires reliable technology, including screening tests with high sensitivity (the ability to identify positive results) and specificity (the ability to identify negative results). In general, resource-poor settings lack trained medical staff or the facilities to offer expensive laboratory tests. In the 1990s, syndromic management of STIs was introduced to address this problem. With this approach, STI diagnosis and treatment is based not on the cause of the disease (aetiology), but on syndromes (groups of signs and symptoms). Treatment is offered that will deal with most, or at least the most serious, aetiological agents causing the syndrome.

Activity 14.1

Can you identify some advantages and disadvantages of treating STIs syndromically?

Feedback

Advantages
- The cost is lower and algorithms are used that can take account of local STI prevalence rates.
- Does not require expensive laboratory testing equipment
- Treatment can start immediately instead of having to wait for laboratory results.

Disadvantages
Syndromic management works better for men than women; urethral discharge is a fairly reliable indicator of an STI in men, but vaginal discharge is a less reliable indicator of an STI (gonorrhoea and Chlamydia) in women, being more often the result of a non-sexually transmitted infection.

Low specificity may mean that some service users end up taking unnecessary medication. This can lead to drug resistance and unnecessary costs, and could cause needless strain on a relationship.

Despite its limitations, syndromic management is still the recommended approach in settings with restricted facilities.

Management also involves supporting those diagnosed with an STI or HIV in notifying their sexual partner(s). The majority of patients are willing to notify their partners but some are reluctant because they feel stigmatized or fear being abused (Alam et al., 2010). Counselling individuals about the partner notification process can improve the outcome of partner referral (Alam et al., 2010).

Prevention of unplanned pregnancy

The provision of contraceptive products should ideally be accompanied by education and counselling to enable service users to make an informed choice, and to support consistent and correct use of the chosen method.

Despite the availability of a wide range of modern low-cost methods, unmet need for contraception is estimated to be high globally (see Chapter 3). Options are often limited, even in high-income settings, and the provider may have a strong influence on choice of method. A survey in the UK found that poor knowledge and attitudes among general practitioners concerning long-acting reversible contraceptive methods (including misconceptions about eligibility and side effects, and concerns about high discontinuation rates) served as barriers to provision (Wellings et al., 2007).

Provision of safe abortion

Abortion is the most frequent clinical procedure undergone by women. If carried out correctly by trained professionals, the procedure is safe and effective. Nevertheless, over 20 million unsafe abortions take place worldwide each year (Shah and Áhman, 2010; see also Chapter 3). This is because women without access to safe abortion often resort to using unskilled providers or use methods without clinical supervision.

Abortions are induced either by surgical removal of the foetus or medically, using pharmaceutical drugs. The latter is feasible and acceptable to both women and providers, and gives women the option to be treated in a less clinical environment, by nurses rather than doctors (Mundle et al., 2007). Good abortion care also involves follow-up services such as the provision of contraceptive counselling (WHO, 2010).

Promotion of sexual health and wellbeing

A key role for sexual health services is the promotion of sexual wellbeing. The aim here is to help individuals and couples experience sex as positive and enjoyable. In particular, individuals and couples experiencing sexual function problems should be offered counselling and medical intervention, if appropriate (see Chapter 5). Unfortunately, this role is often neglected, and sexuality issues are often left out of consultations (Askew and Berer, 2003). In conservative and under-resourced countries, counselling for sexual function problems is rare, and even medical treatment for erectile dysfunction may not be widely available. Little progress has been made in integrating sexual function into general sexual health services. Even in the relatively well-resourced UK health service, only 25% of genito-urinary clinics have a designated service for sexual dysfunction (Green and Goldmeier, 2008).

Other services

Other areas that can fall under the remit of sexual health services include: support for those experiencing sexual violence or coercion, maternal and new-born health, treatment for infertility, reproductive tract cancers, treatment of menstrual disorders, sexual orientation and gender identity issues.

Delivery of services

The mode of service delivery varies across different settings, depending on the social, cultural and political context, the health needs and demands of the population, the available resources, and the existing infrastructure (WHO, 2011).

Activity 14.2

Think about how sexual health services are delivered in your local area. Make a list of the different providers and the services they offer.

Feedback

You may find that you have quite a long list of providers working in a range of contexts. Sexual health services may be provided at four key levels of health care: primary, secondary, tertiary and outreach.

At the primary level, family doctors, genito-urinary medicine clinics, and family planning clinics may provide sexual health services. At secondary and tertiary levels, hospital gynaecologists and urologists may provide abortions and treatment for erectile dysfunction, respectively.

Outreach programmes may be run in schools, youth centres, and prisons as well bringing services to people in rural areas. Such programmes are good at targeting those who are not accessing primary services, particularly those at high-risk of poor sexual health outcomes. Outreach programmes using trained female community workers to bring contraceptive services to the doorstep proved highly effective in Bangladesh during the 1980s (Cleland et al., 2006).

In addition, contraceptive products may be available at commercial outlets such as pharmacies and shops. The private sector has become increasingly involved in the delivery of sexual health services in many countries, often usefully filling gaps left by the public sector (such as treatment for sexual dysfunction). Private providers have been shown to be effective at increasing contraceptive use (Peters et al., 2004). For instance, the sale of oral contraceptives by the pharmaceutical industry via pharmacies contributed significantly to meeting unmet need in Brazil and bringing down the total fertility rate from 6.2% in 1960 to 2.5% in 1996 (Cleland et al., 2006). However, evidence of the impact of the private sector on STI control and treatment is still lacking.

Service use is maximized where potential users have a choice of service type. Some prefer to see their general practitioner or family doctor because they seek continuity of care and familiarity; others prefer greater anonymity. However, for the majority of service users there is no choice and, under these circumstances, the available services need to work especially hard to cater to a wide range of needs.

Service provision globally

Historically, the management of STIs has received little attention. Prior to the 1980s, STI treatment was confined to specialist clinics in hospitals and targeted at men (Askew and Berer, 2003). As a result, STIs were mostly self-treated, with the help of pharmacists, drug sellers, and traditional healers. The detection and management of STIs became a priority after 1980, with the advent of HIV and introduction of syndromic management of STIs. However, even today, services for STIs in many countries are disjointed and disorganized; and they still often do not reach those who are most in need of them (Askew and Berer, 2003). In comparison, over the past few decades, family planning services in most countries have been relatively well funded and supported by high levels of technical expertise (Askew and Berer, 2003); though it is argued that the family-planning agenda has dropped down the list of international development priorities more recently (Cleland et al., 2006).

Changing patterns in the provision of sexual health services can be understood against a backdrop of shifts in funding mechanisms and macro-level policies for health in general. Since the mid-twentieth century, the global health policy debate has witnessed a series of oscillations between vertical and horizontal approaches (Church, 2012). The latter approach – articulated by the Alma Ata Declaration of 1978 – calls for comprehensive primary health care services that address the social determinants of health. Vertical approaches, on the other hand, target specific diseases and tend to arise from political decisions based on the epidemiological, socio-economic, and/or political importance of a disease (Criel et al., 1997). Although their drawbacks were identified as long ago as the 1960s – Alma Ata was partly a response to these drawbacks – vertical programmes have grown in number during the last few decades (Church, 2012), in part because they are favoured by international donors. They have had some success in controlling specific diseases (such as small pox) and addressing needs of specific populations (such as mothers and children) (Church, 2012). Some argue that vertical programmes impede governments from building strong health systems, and limit opportunities for integrating services. Others point to evidence that funding for vertical interventions has been used to strengthen existing health services and argue for a synergy of vertical and horizontal approaches (Church, 2012). This approach has been termed 'diagonal' health financing (Ooms et al., 2008).

Service integration: 'one-stop shops'

Sexual health needs are commonly related; outcomes such as pregnancy and STIs both result from the same cause (unprotected sex). And many adverse sexual health outcomes (such as sexual violence and unplanned pregnancy) share similar root causes, including poverty, social marginalization, and lack of access to services (Church, 2012). Although the majority of HIV infections are transmitted sexually, around 10% are associated with pregnancy, childbirth, and breast-feeding. There are clear benefits to educating service users about pregnancy prevention and STI prevention at the same time. These factors provide a strong *a priori* rationale for integrating reproductive health services and STI services.

This logic provided the impetus for the call, at the International Conference on Population and Development (ICPD) in Cairo in 1994, to institute comprehensive sexual and reproductive health services (Church and Mayhew, 2009). However, during the 1990s, the considerable challenges of integrating STI management into reproductive health services became apparent, in particular the challenge of providing adequate STI diagnosis and treatment within traditional family planning services (Church and Mayhew, 2009). For services in resource-poor settings with limited budgets and poorly trained staff, the obstacles to adding a new speciality to their existing repertoire often proved insurmountable. In addition, vertical programmes for HIV are sometimes implemented in ways that hinder integration (Mayhew et al., 2005). There have been renewed efforts at integration more recently, driven by the need to address the reproductive and sexual health needs of people living with AIDS, as well as recognition of the benefits of providing HIV testing and treatment to people attending reproductive health care services (Church and Mayhew, 2009).

Essentially, integration implies 'having multi-purpose staff, a multi-purpose team and clinic, or an effective referral mechanism to address a range of different health care needs' (Church, 2012).

Integration can take place at different levels:

- at the point of service delivery (the one-stop shop approach);
- across health services (such as linked family planning and genito-urinary medicine services);
- with other sectors and agencies (such as schools and non-government organizations);
- at a national policy, planning, and development level.

There is not always agreement about how best to integrate services in practice (French et al., 2006). In general, the approach taken will depend on local needs, existing infrastructure and resources, and the policy context. It may not be feasible or appropriate to set up a one-stop shop service, particularly in areas that are already under-staffed and have limited resources. However, integration strategies may make effective use of the existing service infrastructure, for instance by adding an additional speciality (STI prevention) to an existing service (family planning). Experience from both high STI prevalence countries (Kenya and Zimbabwe) and low prevalence countries (Indonesia) suggests that such an approach is feasible as long as staff are well prepared and trained, and have non-judgemental attitudes (Church, 2012). Elsewhere (e.g. Haiti and Uganda), there has been some success at integrating reproductive health services into existing HIV services. An integrated mindset among staff working in services is as important as facilities and resources. This implies that staff members take opportunities to reach people not accessing other types of sexual health service. For instance, men rarely visit family planning services, but they do visit STI services and the staff there may take the opportunity to discuss contraception with them.

A recent review concluded that integrated services are cost-effective, acceptable to clients, can increase access to constituent services, and reduce HIV-related stigma in clinics (Church and Mayhew, 2009). However, the evidence that reproductive health services can reach men, as well as the evidence for their impact on health outcomes, is inconclusive (Church and Mayhew, 2009).

Activity 14.3

What might be the potential advantages and disadvantages of one-stop shops?

Feedback

The advantages and disadvantages are summarized in Table 14.1.

Table 14.1 Potential advantages and disadvantages of 'one-stop shops'

Perspective	Advantages	Disadvantages
Public health	• Health needs related: clients at risk of STIs may also be at risk of unplanned pregnancy, and vice versa • Follow-up is likely to be more efficient, since fewer clients will be lost through referral	• Capacity to treat one condition may be reduced by the need to treat several • The objectives of the different specialities may be divergent (e.g. promotion of condoms for STI prevention may conflict with need for optimal contraceptive effectiveness)
Users	• One-stop shops may be more convenient, less complicated, and less time-consuming • The reason for the visit may be less obvious to others • Integration normalizes sexual health and offers a holistic approach	• Some services may be lost because of centralization • Stigma may attend some services more than others; those wanting contraceptive services may prefer not to be associated with STIs • Clients wanting a specialist service may miss a sense of service identity
Staff	• Job satisfaction may be improved through greater autonomy • Professional education and career opportunities are likely to be improved	• Loyalty to, and a sense of professional identity with, a specialty may be lost • Opportunities for increasing remuneration with skill level may be compromised
Logistics	• Convenience • One set of case notes/integrated technology	• Lack of space • Data collection systems in the different specialties may not be compatible
Cost	• Greater efficiency by avoiding duplication, e.g. shared staff, equipment, and overheads	• High set-up costs, including staff training • Possibility of inequities in funding across different specialities

Barriers to sexual health care

Barriers to sexual health care services fall into several categories and relate to availability, accessibility, acceptability, and equity. These are described below, together with possible ways in which they might be addressed.

Availability

The availability of services may be sub-optimal because of a lack of resources and/or a lack of political will. Funding problems are likely to be compounded by political resistance in the case of poorer countries, where sexual health services may be seen as a low priority for limited resources. But political obstacles to provision have beset some of the richest countries in the world. In 2012, this was evident in the furore over provision of abortion and family planning in the USA.

Although services may be available in theory, in practice the selective systems they operate may bar some categories of users. In countries in which sexual behaviour is tightly restricted, services may not be accessible to specific groups. In some areas of Pakistan, family planning services are not available to unmarried women. In India, where strong social norms prohibit premarital sex, the negative attitudes of service providers as well as reluctance to report being sexually active limit access by unmarried youth (Collumbien et al., 2011). In countries where homosexuality is illegal and carries harsh penalties, services may not be available to men who have sex with men.

A range of interventions may be required to address structural influences on service availability (Chapter 10). These include advocacy work to challenge restrictive norms and promote sexual health rights, as well as lobbying for changes to the law. Where resources limit supply, interventions might include lobbying politically for better funding or improved configuration of services, as well as providing training and support to alternative providers (such as non-governmental organizations or the private sector) to fill gaps in public provision of services. India's recent national strategies to address the sexual and reproductive health needs of youth have led to better availability of services to targeted groups, and may have helped to weaken the traditional belief that fertility should be demonstrated soon after marriage (Collumbien et al., 2011).

Accessibility

Services may be available, but under-utilized. The barriers that prevent potential users from accessing sexual health services have been well documented. Although much of the research concerns young people as service users, many of the barriers they face are relevant to adults too, particularly those whose sexual behaviour does not conform to social norms. Although a number of initiatives are recommended by WHO with respect to services for young people, few have been rigorously assessed via controlled experiments (Tylee et al., 2007).

Accessibility depends on a range of factors, including convenience, level of publicity, and cost. Inconvenience is a major barrier to service use. Convenience implies practical opening hours, easy attendance with short waiting times (whether via an appointment system or drop-in service), swift referral, and easily accessible locations. For example, services for young people need to be open outside of school or college hours, and services attended by young mothers need to be child-friendly. Services may be inaccessible simply because potential service users are not aware that they exist.

Interventions to improve accessibility can impact not only on individual but also population sexual health. For example, at the population level, it has been demonstrated that teenage pregnancy rates decline when contraception is more readily available to young people (Santelli et al., 2007). Modern technology is increasingly being used by service providers and has the potential to improve accessibility. Recently, this has included text messaging and online services for sexual health promotion, for partner notification, and for appointment reminders (Lim et al., 2008). The benefits include low cost, good accessibility, and the ability to reach many people.

Costs of consultations, medicines, and condoms can act as a barrier to access for some sub-populations. Voucher scheme programmes, designed to overcome this barrier, are gaining in popularity. These schemes involve free or heavily subsidized vouchers distributed to potential service users. Providers are then reimbursed for treating voucher-bearing service users. A review of these programmes in developing countries found they had a positive effect on utilization of sexual health services, although their cost-effectiveness and health impact at a population level require further research (Bellows et al., 2011).

In family planning recently, accessibility has been increased by dispensing with unnecessary constraints and rules regarding medical practice, such as the need to have written consent from a husband or obliging women to return for an excessive number of follow-up visits (Cleland et al., 2006). Increasingly, research has shown that many of the core procedures, such as fitting an intrauterine device, can be undertaken by paramedics and need not require medical doctors.

Acceptability

For those whose sexual behaviour does not comply with the moral codes of their social environment (e.g. sexually active and unmarried young people, men who have sex with men, sex workers), acceptability in terms of quality of service provision is a key issue.

Service integration may impact on acceptability for certain groups of clients. For instance, where STI prevention services have been integrated into family planning clinics, men, young people, and sex workers may feel uncomfortable attending 'women-focused' reproductive health centres (Church, 2012).

A predominant fear concerns confidentiality. Young people, for instance, may fear being recognized in a clinic or their parents finding out (whether through the health worker or another way). For instance, a study in rural Uganda found that young people would rather pay to visit informal and traditional healers because they offered a level of confidentiality and privacy that they felt was lacking in public services (Kiapi-Iwa and Hart, 2004). To address these concerns, services require comprehensive confidentiality policies, and where possible users should be seen without other family members or partners present.

Another barrier to service provision is the anticipation of unfriendly and judgemental staff and of unpleasant and embarrassing procedures. Fears about disapproval are sometimes realized. During a simulated client study in Dakar, Senegal, young people posing as clients were given unsolicited advice (for example, on the need to abstain from sex until marriage) at the same time as being given information on family planning. Of the six clients who requested contraceptives, none was given any, and one (who was about to marry) was told to return with evidence of permission from her future husband (Katz and Naré, 2002).

A priority during history-taking and examination is to help the service user to feel welcomed and comfortable. Empathic body language, and clear and non-judgemental language is key to this process (see Chapter 11). Good sexual histories go beyond the measurement of exposure to risk – they also involve discussion of the social context. For instance, adolescents who have not told their parents that they are sexually active may not want to take any contraceptive supplies (such as pill packets) home with them and a good healthcare worker will be sensitive to these concerns. Ideally, sexual histories would include questions about sexual function or difficulties in order to pick up any unmet need. Privacy is important, particularly during physical examinations. Being seen by a healthcare worker of the same gender can reduce anxiety, but this is not always possible.

Informed consent procedures – in which screening tests, procedures, examinations, and treatment are clearly explained before being administered – can help to alleviate fears. Consent is 'informed' only if service users understand what will happen, the likely outcomes and the associated risks. Informed consent also implies that service users understand their options and are able to make informed decisions about their care as appropriate.

For all service users, quality of care impacts greatly on acceptability. Aspects of quality include competent diagnosis and clinical management, availability of effective medicines, well-equipped and clean examination rooms, and short waiting times.

With regard to quality, a key intervention is regular training for staff, to improve professional practice. Training should also address issues such as judgemental attitudes, reluctance to raise issues of sexuality and pleasure, and poor communication strategies (see Chapter 11).

For some potential users, it is the products themselves that are unacceptable rather than the ways in which services are delivered. For instance, in some areas of sub-Saharan Africa, and in strongly Catholic countries, the idea of contraception to limit family size is still considered unacceptable. Strategies to create a climate supportive of modern family planning need to involve mass media approaches as well as the creation of broad coalitions between religious and traditional leaders, professional groups, and other key sectors of society (Cleland et al., 2006). Social marketing can also be used to create demand for products (see Chapter 12).

Equity

Pricing systems and differences in the scope of health insurance schemes can make services inaccessible to poorer people but not the rich. The configuration and location of services may make them more accessible to those in urban areas compared with those in rural areas. For those who are poor and living rurally, even the cost of transportation to clinic can be prohibitive.

Interventions to address issues of equity involve policies and practices that explicitly seek to remove obstacles to use by those traditionally excluded from the service. Such interventions might include establishing an outreach programme and addressing staff attitudes to excluded groups via additional training. Introducing more equitable payment systems is also important. A benefit of the voucher scheme programmes mentioned above is that they can be targeted at low-income or high-risk populations.

Summary

Sexual health services have a wide remit, including prevention and control of STIs and HIV, prevention of unplanned pregnancy, provision of safe abortion, and promotion of sexual health. Services may be configured in a variety of ways but often service users have complex needs and an integrated approach may be beneficial. Many clients are excluded from services; barriers to service use relate to availability, accessibility, acceptability, and equity. Interventions to address these barriers centre on improving the availability of services relative to the needs of the population, and training staff to improve quality and promote positive values and attitudes. Structural interventions may be required to address barriers arising from stigma and from legal restrictions on the provision of services.

References

Alam N, Chamot E, Vermund SH, Streatfield K and Kristensen S (2010) Partner notification for sexually transmitted infections in developing countries: a systematic review, *BMC Public Health*, 10: 19.

Askew I and Berer M (2003) The contribution of sexual and reproductive health services in the fight against HIV/AIDS: a review, *Reproductive Health Matters*, 11(22): 51–73.

Bellows NM, Bellows BW and Warren C (2011) The use of vouchers for reproductive health services in developing countries: systematic review, *Tropical Medicine and International Health*, 16(1): 84–96.

Church K (2012) Integrating STI prevention, care and treatment with other sexual and reproductive health services, in S. Gupta and B. Kumar (eds.) *Sexually Transmitted Infections*, 2nd edn. New Delhi: Eslevier.

Church K and Mayhew SH (2009) Integration of STI and HIV prevention, care and treatment into family planning services: a review of the literature, *Studies in Family Planning*, 40(3): 171–86.

Cleland J, Berstein MS, Ezeh A, Faundes A, Glasier A and Innis J (2006) Family planning: the unfinished agenda, *Lancet*, 368(9549): 1810–27.

Collumbien M, Mishra M and Blackmore C (2011) Youth-friendly services in two rural districts of West Bengal and Jharkhand, India: definite progress, a long way to go, *Reproductive Health Matters*, 19(37): 174–83.

Criel B, De Brouwere V and Dugas S (1997) *Integration of Vertical Programmes in Multi-function Health Services*. Antwerp: ITG Press.

French RS, Coope CM, Graham A, Gerressu M, Salisbury C, Stephenson JM et al. (2006) One stop shop versus collaborative integration: what is the best way of delivering sexual health services?, *Sexually Transmitted Infections*, 82: 202–6.

Green P and Goldmeier D (2008) Sexual dysfunction service provision in UK genitourinary medicine clinics in 2007, *International Journal of STD and AIDS*, 19(1): 30–3.

Katz K and Naré C (2002) Reproductive health knowledge and use of services among young adults in Dakar, Senegal, *Journal of Biosocial Science*, 34: 215–31.

Kiapi-Iwa L and Hart GJ (2004) The sexual and reproductive health of young people in Adjumani district, Uganda: qualitative study of the role of formal, informal and traditional health providers, *AIDS Care*, 16(3): 339–47.

Lim MSC, Hocking JS, Hellard ME and Aitken CK (2008) SMS STI: a review of the uses of mobile phone text messaging in sexual health, *International Journal of STD and AIDS*, 19: 287–90.

Mayhew SH, Walt G, Lush L and Cleland J (2005) Donor agencies' involvement in reproductive health: saying one thing and doing another?, *International Journal of Health Services*, 35: 24–9.

Medical Foundation for AIDS and Sexual Health (MedFash) (2005) *Recommended Standards for Sexual Health Services*. London: Department of Health. Available at: http://www.medfash.org.uk/publications/documents/Recommended_standards_for_sexual_health_services.pdf (accessed 8 July 2011).

Mundle S, Elul B, Anand A and Kalyanwala S (2007) Increasing access to safe abortion in rural India: experiences to safe abortion in a primary health center, *Contraception*, 76(1): 66–70.

Ooms G, Van Damme W, Baker BK, Zeitz P and Schrecker T (2008) The 'diagonal' approach to Global Fund financing: a cure for the broader malaise of health systems?, *Globalization and Health*, 4: 6.

Peters DH, Mirchandani GC and Hansen PM (2004) Strategies for engaging the private sector in sexual and reproductive health: how effective are they?, *Health Policy and Planning*, 19(1): i15–i21.

Santelli JS, Lindberg LD, Finer LB and Singh S (2007) Explaining recent declines in adolescent pregnancy in the United States: the contribution of abstinence and improved contraceptive use, *American Journal of Public Health*, 97(1): 150–6.

Shah I and Áhman E (2010) Unsafe abortion in 2008: global and regional levels and trends, *Reproductive Health Matters*, 18(36): 90–101.

Tylee A, Haller DM, Graham T, Churchill R and Sanci LA (2007) Youth-friendly primary-care services: how are we doing and what more needs to be done?, *Lancet*, 369(9572): 1565–73.

Wellings K, Zhihong Z, Krentel A, Barraett G and Glasier A (2007) Attitudes towards long-acting reversible methods in general practice in the UK, *Contraception*, 76(3): 208–14.

World Health Organization (WHO) (2007) *Global Strategy for the Prevention and Control of Sexually Transmitted Infections, 2006–2015 – Breaking the Chain of Transmission*. Geneva: WHO. Available at: http://whqlibdoc.who.int/publications/2007/9789241563475_eng.pdf (accessed 17 June 2011).

World Health Organization (WHO) (2010) *Packages of Interventions for Family Planning, Safe Abortion Care, Maternal, Newborn and Child Health*. Geneva: WHO. Available at: http://whqlibdoc.who.int/hq/2010/WHO_FCH_10.06_eng.pdf (accessed 17 June 2011).

World Health Organization (WHO) (2011) *Quality of Care in the Provision of Sexual and Reproductive Health Services*. Geneva: WHO.

Further reading

World Health Organization (WHO) (2010) *Developing Sexual Health Programmes: A Framework for Action*. Geneva: WHO.

PART 5

Measuring and assessing sexual health status

Researching sexual behaviour

Kaye Wellings and Martine Collumbien

Overview

Previous chapters in this book have shown that robust data on sexual behaviour are a cornerstone of efforts to improve sexual health. In this chapter, we explore some approaches to, and challenges for, research into sexual behaviour. We examine sources of possible bias, their implications for interpreting results, and ways of improving the quality of data.

Learning outcomes

After reading this chapter, you will be able to:

- Describe approaches to, and challenges for, research into sexual behaviour
- Understand sources of possible bias and their implications for interpreting data
- Identify ways in which data quality can be improved

Key terms

Generalizability: The extent to which the findings of a study can be reliably extrapolated from the participants to a broader population represented by the sample.

Participation bias: Error arising from systematic differences in the behaviour of those people in the selected sample who agree to participate compared with those in the selected sample who do not agree to take part.

Reliability: The extent to which measurements taken at different time points remain stable and consistent.

Reporting bias: Error arising from differences between the accounts given by study participants and their actual experience.

Validity: The extent to which a research instrument measures what it sets out to measure.

Introduction

Reliable information about sexual behaviour is essential to the design and assessment of interventions to improve sexual health, to an understanding of the aetiology of sexual ill health, and to the development of appropriately targeted sexual health services. An understanding of trends and patterns in sexual behaviour is essential to the design of effective interventions aimed at improving sexual health status and to assessing progress towards this goal. Data from comparative studies are vital in guiding the effective targeting and tailoring of interventions to specific social groups and contexts. Importantly, too, empirical evidence is needed to correct myths in public perception of behaviours.

Challenges for research

Sexual behaviours are personal and for the most part take place in private and so possibilities for direct observation are limited. There are also fewer opportunities for triangulation of data than there are for behaviours such as smoking and drinking, where consumption can be measured through sales figures, for example.

Many behaviours of interest in a public health context are socially disapproved of and some are illegal. Some involve people who are hard to reach, remain hidden or wary of taking part in research. This has consequences for the quality of data collected. Behaviours that are strongly socially sanctioned are more prone to a social desirability effect, the tendency to respond according to a perception of what is socially acceptable. It also has consequences for whether research is conducted at all. Researchers in the field of sexual conduct have habitually met with resistance and hostility. Alfred Kinsey, working in the mid-twentieth century, was threatened with dismissal for his groundbreaking studies of sexual behaviour. Even in the 1980s, when data were urgently needed in the context of the HIV epidemic, the British National Survey of Sexual Attitudes and Lifestyles (Natsal) was vetoed by the then Prime Minister, Mrs. Thatcher, as likely to be intrusive and a waste of money. It was rescued by funding from the Wellcome Trust (Wellings et al., 1990).

How is sexual behaviour researched?

Historically, approaches to the study of sexual behaviour have reflected changing perspectives on the subject. In the nineteenth century, the focus was on pathology, on the medical and psychiatric investigation of sexual disorders, and most studies were of clinically 'deviant' cases. The mid-twentieth century was marked by the pioneering surveys of Alfred Kinsey in the USA (Kinsey et al., 1948, 1953). In the late 1960s, Masters and Johnson conducted studies of sexual response, in which participants were observed in laboratory conditions, and their physiological reaction to sexual stimuli measured (Masters and Johnson, 1966).

Of greatest interest in a contemporary public health context are preferences and patterns of behaviour, how they vary with social group, and what the implications are for sexual health status. These areas rely largely on individual reports – usually retrospective – elicited typically through survey work or in-depth studies.

Community-based surveys are the stock-in-trade for measuring the prevalence of behaviours. Cross-sectional surveys provide a snapshot in time. They allow trends to be described using birth cohort analysis, but only for activities that occur once in a lifetime such as first sex. Repeat cross-sectional surveys offer an improvement in this respect, but longitudinal studies are the ideal method for monitoring behaviour over time, despite problems of attrition.

Hard to reach groups

For many behaviours of interest to sexual health researchers, such as injecting drug use, sex work, and intimate partner violence, representative general population surveys may not be appropriate. Those who practise such behaviours are often missing from conventional sampling frames; their willingness to participate may be lower; and, since they comprise only small fractions of the population, general samples would in any case yield insufficient numbers of participants to sustain statistical analysis.

For hard to reach groups, focused studies are more appropriate, using purposive or convenience sampling strategies, including snowballing techniques, recruitment from specific settings (such as health services and commercial venues), and respondent-driven sampling. Success has been achieved by working with outreach and rehabilitation schemes, by enrolling members of the study community in the research team, and by providing reciprocal benefits where possible (Fenton et al., 2001).

Choice of data collection method

Face-to-face personal interviews, using fully scheduled and structured questionnaires, remain the most common method of collecting data on sexual behaviour. There is, however, some scepticism as to whether this is the best method of facilitating personal disclosure (Cleland et al., 2004). This aim may be best achieved by unstructured interviews, though these lend themselves less readily to provision of, for example, prevalence estimates. Telephone interviews are cheaper, but offer no advantages to face-to-face methods in terms of enhancing disclosure, since they lack possibilities for using aids such as show cards. They are also prone to an 'eavesdropper' effect as other household members may be listening in. They have, however, been used successfully in a number or surveys, including the French national sexual behaviour surveys (ACSF) (Bajos and Spira, 1992).

Computer-assisted techniques, including CAPI (Computer-Assisted Personal Interviews), CASI (Computer-Assisted Self Interviews), and CATI (Computer-Assisted Telephone Interviews), represent important methodological advances. These methods allow responses to be keyed directly into computers. Skips and routing can be automatically programmed, enhancing confidentiality and facilitating self-correction by respondents, and thus improving the quality of the data. Computer-assisted techniques are expensive and in resource-poor countries this is a major drawback. Comparable results have been experienced by use of 'low-tech' solutions, including the use of informal confidential voting interviews (ICVI), in which answers to questions are anonymously 'posted' into boxes (Gregson et al., 2004). Combinations of self-completion and interviewer techniques are used in many large surveys, combining the benefits of face-to-face interviews with the privacy of self-completion.

Qualitative research

Survey research has a vital role in the measurement of sexual behaviour, particularly in yielding prevalence estimates, and has provided much of the empirical basis for sexual and reproductive health programme design, monitoring, and evaluation. Survey methods, however, are of limited value in understanding the complexity of people's sexual lifestyles, the meanings sexual behaviours have for them, and their motivations for behaving in particular ways. Qualitative research methods are often used to complement quantitative methods – in the design of questionnaires, in illuminating associations found in quantitative analysis, and in triangulating data. But perhaps the greatest value of qualitative methods lies in their potential to explore and probe more deeply into people's accounts of sexual practices and partnerships than survey methods allow (Marston and King, 2006).

Qualitative studies make an essential contribution to our understanding of the significance of sexual behaviours for individuals and of the nature of the social context in which they take place. Since such methods allow the exploration of meanings, they perform better in terms of validity than do survey methods, and so are also essential to the design of survey research instruments and to the triangulation of results from quantitative research (Mitchell et al., 2007). Again, most are retrospective but where the use of sexual diaries is appropriate, prospective collection of data is possible, minimizing problems associated with long-term recall and so improving the quality of data.

Combining behavioural and biomedical measures

A limitation of most sexual health research in the past has been the lack of biological data, for example, on infection, and on hormonal and pregnancy status. Conducted separately, social science research and clinical surveillance both have shortcomings. A limitation of social research is its reliance on self-reports, which correlate poorly with laboratory evidence, while surveillance systems exclude people diagnosed outside of health services, and so provide no measure of the burden of untreated sexual ill health in the community.

Important technological developments, including new non-invasive techniques for measuring STI infection and hormonal status, are beginning to facilitate a fusion of disciplinary perspectives. As community-based methods for collecting specimens become cheaper and less intrusive, the inclusion of biological markers in large-scale studies has become more justifiable and feasible. As a result, partnerships between clinical, epidemiological, and social scientists have increased. This has provided opportunities for studying the relation between behavioural and biomedical markers. It has also facilitated the triangulation of results to assess the validity of reported data (Glynn et al., 2011).

Introducing bias

Bias occurs when the reported behaviour of those taking part in a study differs from that of the population the sample was chosen to represent, in ways that are important to the research. All research reliant on self-reports is susceptible to bias, and some take the view that studies with a focus on sexual behaviour suffer no more in this respect than studies of other sensitive topics, such as personal income, voting patterns, and smoking. But because sexual behaviour is so heavily socially regulated and circumscribed (Chapter 1), its empirical study may be especially prone to bias. Hence the need for greater vigilance and precautionary measures.

Bias can be introduced at any stage of a study, from sample selection to questionnaire design or administration. It may arise through *participation bias*, where the reluctance of participants to take part because of the subject matter, or failure to reach them, can lead to problems of *generalizability*. Alternatively, it may arise through *reporting bias*, where people may neglect to answer questions because they are sensitive or difficult to understand, or provide responses that do not accurately reflect their experience, or are unstable (changing from one time to the next), leading to problems of *validity* and *reliability*.

Participation bias

Participation bias describes error arising from differences in the behaviour of those who agree to participate in a study compared with those who do not. It is a problem that particularly besets studies that use volunteer samples. Alfred Kinsey, for example, famously recruited his sample from his lecture audiences, from prison populations, and the armed forces. Impressive though the studies were, they provided no guarantee of the representativeness of the sample in terms of behavioural characteristics. Compared with those randomly recruited from the general population, volunteers may be more, or less, sexually adventurous or sensation-seeking or liberal in their views, but they cannot be relied upon to be typical of the mass of the population about whom information is needed. Random probability sampling is the more sophisticated approach, and offers considerably greater promise in obtaining a representative sample. Using sampling frames such as electoral registers, postcode address files, and telephone directories, such techniques in theory give every member of the population an equal chance of being recruited. Yet even they may underrepresent certain groups, such as the homeless, those without a phone, and the most mobile members of society. In many countries, such sampling frames simply do not exist.

All studies are essentially 'voluntary' at the point of contact, since people cannot be coerced into taking part. Achieving good response rates is therefore essential to ensure that the sample is as representative as possible and that the findings can be generalized to the wider population. Even well-designed studies rarely achieve response rates in excess of 70%, although higher response rates are often achieved in developing countries. Response rates are generally lower among men than women, and among those who are older and have less education. Although these differences can be corrected by weighting the sample, they may affect estimates if non-participation is related to sexual behaviours.

Reporting bias

A number of factors are likely to introduce reporting bias. Because sexual behaviour is most commonly studied retrospectively, recall of behaviours may be a problem. Recall difficulties are more marked in relation to frequency (e.g. numbers of occasions of sex in a particular period) than incidence (such as first sexual intercourse). In general, recall diminishes with time since occurrence but increases with salience (events like first intercourse are for most people easy to remember). More difficult to remember are events that accumulate over a long period of time, such as numbers of sexual partners, particularly for those with large numbers. Since we continuously interpret and reinterpret the events of our lives, retrospectively, recall is likely to impact on reliability. Reporting bias may also be introduced as a result of questions being misunderstood or interpreted in ways other than intended.

The interviewer may also introduce bias. Face-to-face interviews have advantages in enabling interviewers to explain the rationale and format of a survey, and to provide motivation, clarification, and support; but they also have the capacity to influence what is reported and how. The evidence is that people are more comfortable reporting on matters of sexual behaviour to a woman than to a man.

Identifying bias and interpreting data: bridging the gap between what people do and say

Two important questions for sexual behaviour research are: 'How can we detect bias?' and 'How can we interpret it?' We present below two examples illustrating gender differences in responses – possibly the most common bias in studies of sexual behaviour. Many studies have found major, and implausible, discrepancies in reporting of sexual practices and partnerships.

Example 1: Reporting age at first intercourse

Figure 15.1 shows data on age at onset of heterosexual intercourse from two repeat cross-sectional Natsal surveys, carried out in 1990 and 2000 in Britain. The data are plotted by birth dates, and show year moving averages. They represent the proportion

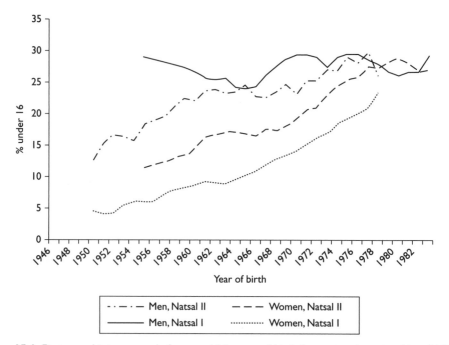

Figure 15.1 First sexual intercourse before age 16 by year of birth for men and women: Natsal I (1990) and Natsal II (2000) moving averages

Source: Copas et al. (2002)

of men and women in successive birth cohorts who reported first sexual intercourse occurring before age 16 years. Of interest is the change over time in this proportion. Differences in reports between two or more time points may reflect:

- *A change in the method of data collection used*: Using different methods of gathering data at different time points; for example, replacing pen and paper with computer-assisted interviews may alter reporting and the data may reflect this.
- *A change in the social climate*: Shifts in the social norms governing behaviour may be reflected in increased ease of reporting as well as a change in the behaviour itself.
- *Variations in the sample*: The composition of the sample used in the survey reported at earlier time points differs from that of the later survey sample.
- *A true change in behaviour*: A genuine change in behaviour has occurred between the time points.

A common birth cohort, of men and women, born between 1950 and 1984, is represented in the random probability samples in both the Natsal I (1990) and the Natsal II (2000) surveys. We could thus expect their responses to questions about events in early life to be the same in both studies. For example, the proportion of women born in the mid-1950s reporting first intercourse before 16 should be the same whether they were reporting in 1990 or 2000. This is not the case (Figure 15.1). The proportion of women reporting first sex before 16 steadily increases with successive birth cohorts in both surveys. But the proportion doing so in Natsal II in 2000 (represented by the dashed line) is some 5–10% higher than the proportion doing so in Natsal I in 1990 (the dotted line). Looking at the Natsal 2000 data for men (solid line), we see little change over time. This contrasts with the Natsal 1990 data (dot-dash line), which show a steady increase over time in the proportion of men sexually active before age 16, suggesting that the apparent increase in the proportion of men having sex before age 16 may have been largely due to a reporting bias.

We can look at this same phenomenon in Uganda, using data from a random probability DHS survey (Slaymaker et al., 2009). In Figure 15.2, the data from repeat demographic and health surveys (DHS) carried out in 1995 and 2001 have again been plotted to examine time trends, comparing men and women in each survey representing the same birth cohorts.

Comparing the older with the younger age groups in the sample, this time we see a slight *decrease* over time in the proportion of women who had sex before age 15

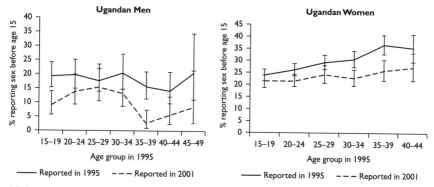

Figure 15.2 Age at first sex in Uganda

in the 1995 survey, a trend that is less marked in the later, 2001 survey. There is no consistent trend for men. But the proportion of both men and women who reported first sex having occurred before age 15 was, *in each comparable age group*, lower in 2001 than it was in 1995. The trend in Uganda has been towards later sex, in contrast to the trend in Britain, which has been towards earlier sex. Yet within that trend, Ugandan women of all ages were more likely to report early sex in the first study, compared with the second, later study, while for British women the reverse was true.

Activity 15.2

To what extent might these data represent real changes over time, and to what extent might they represent a reporting bias? It is important to try to assess which is the case, since public health strategies will be guided by these data.

Looking at Figures 15.1 and 15.2:

- Which of the explanations set out on page 181 best explain the data?
- To what extent is there evidence for bias in these data?
- Is this likely to be reporting bias or a participation bias?
- What might explain the contrast in effects in Britain and Uganda?

Feedback

- *Change in the composition of the sample?* Both the Natsal and the DHS surveys use random probability samples, so we would not expect the composition to have changed greatly over time unless the response rate changed, and it did not.
- *Change in data collection method?* The data collection method used in the two DHS surveys remained the same. In the Natsal II survey in 2000, CAPI and CASI replaced the pencil and paper methods used in Natsal I in 1990, but an experimental study carried out by the researchers revealed that reporting was not significantly affected.
- *Real change or reporting bias?* In the British data, we see a higher proportion of women in every age cohort reporting early sex in 2000 than in 1990. Since these women represent the same age cohorts, this can only be interpreted as a reporting bias, and may reflect a softening of attitudes towards teenage sex, particularly for women, during that period, making reporting easier. In Uganda, an opposite trend is observed, whereby women in the common age cohorts were less likely to report early sex in 2001 than they were in 1995, possibly reflecting less tolerance towards early sex, in the wake of abstinence campaigns, again a reporting bias.

The reporting bias does not, however, explain all the difference, in either case. We also see a *real* increase over time in the rate of first sex before 16 in Britain. In contrast, in Uganda, we see a *real* decrease in the rate of first sex before age 15, possibly reflecting the trend towards later marriage in a country in which first sexual intercourse in most cases occurs between husband and wife.

Example 2: Reporting numbers of sexual partners

Insights into bias can also be gained from comparing differences between countries. In a closed population with a balanced sex ratio, the mean number of partners reported over a defined period should be the same for men and women. Yet in nearly all surveys, men consistently report larger numbers of partners. There are several plausible explanations. This could be because men are having sex with women in age groups or geographical areas not included in the survey sample, or that men are having sex with women with large numbers of partners, such as sex workers, who are under-represented in the sample. Alternatively, it could be that women are defining sex differently to men, or using different strategies to count their partners, or that men are over-reporting and/or women are under-reporting. In other words, what we see in the data is a reporting bias.

In Figure 15.3, sexual behaviour data have been superimposed onto data relating to the age structure in three countries for which sexual behaviour data are available (Wellings et al., 2006). The difference in reporting between men and women is apparent in all the graphs, but the scale of the differences varies between countries. In Britain, the typical features of developed countries can be seen, a symmetrical age structure and considerable gender equality. The number of men reporting more than one sexual partner in the past year is only slightly higher than among women, in each of the age groups.

In Uganda, for both sexes, the proportion reporting multiple partnerships is smaller than in Britain, yet more men than women report multiple partnerships, in every age group. In Brazil, the gender difference is more marked; the number of men reporting multiple partners far outnumbers the number of women doing so.

Activity 15.3

Looking at Figure 15.3:

• How might we explain these patterns?
• Is the explanation likely to be the same in every country?

Feedback

Figure 15.3 shows that the explanation for the differences in reporting between the sexes may vary from place to place. In countries like Britain, with greater gender equality and a symmetrical age structure, the numbers of men and women reporting more than one partner in the past year are similar. In Uganda and Brazil, they are not.

Are the women under-reporting and the men over-reporting in Uganda and Brazil? Not necessarily. Uganda has a markedly pyramidal age structure, with a high proportion of young people in the population. Given the high proportion of men in the youngest age group who reported celibacy in the last year, it is perfectly possible for the men in older age groups to draw their additional partners from the pool of younger, reportedly monogamous, women. In Brazil, the gender disparity in reporting of multiple partners is not explained by the age structure, and it is difficult to avoid the conclusion that men may be 'bragging'. In countries with a 'macho' culture, men may over-report, and women under-report, numbers of sexual partners.

So again, we see a combination of bias and real differences in time, and between countries. Even the bias tells us something about the changing climate, and understanding bias can be helpful. Effective interventions in Uganda, for example, will need to address the phenomenon of 'sugar daddies', while in Brazil they will need to take account of the macho culture.

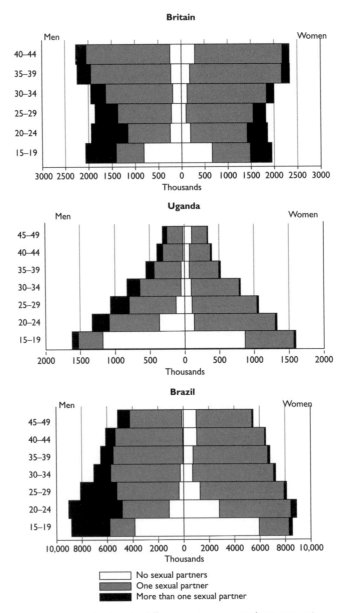

Figure 15.3 Patterns of sexual behaviour in different age groups in three countries

Addressing bias

Although interesting, no amount of *ex post facto* analysis will succeed in improving the quality of the data once collected. It is much better to employ preventive strategies aimed at safeguarding reporting and participation prospectively, at every stage of study development. The need for reliable data on sexual behaviour has provided the impetus for extensive efforts to address the problems of measurement error and bias: to improve the methods used to reach people; to encourage them to take part in research; and to ensure that they are able to give accounts that bear relation to the perceived reality of their lives. Strategies for reducing participation and reporting bias are summarized separately below, but efforts to limit participation bias will often have an impact on reporting bias, and vice versa.

Reducing participation bias: how can people be encouraged to take part?

Since refusal is most likely at the point of initial contact or invitation, many of the following strategies should be introduced at the earliest stage possible in the study.

Men and women may be more inclined to take part if:

- *Confidentiality and anonymity is assured*: this should be underscored in all participant literature relating to the research, including information sheets and consent forms, and the procedures by which it will be safeguarded should be fully described.
- *The importance of the data is fully appreciated*: the public health importance of the study should be explained and the broader benefits of the data emphasized.
- *The calibre, credentials, and integrity of the researchers are evident*: potential participants are more likely to give their time to bona fide academic and social researchers for the public good, than to commercial and media agencies for private gain.
- *Incentives (or rewards) are provided*: where once researchers were wary of influencing the research process by giving incentives, it is now accepted that the time, effort, and contribution of participants should be recognized.
- *Tenacious efforts are made to keep them in the sample*: including respondent call-backs, re-issues to a different interviewer, re-invitations to take part, and postal reminders.

Reducing reporting bias: how can we enable respondents to give authentic accounts?

The term 'authentic' account is preferable to 'honest' or 'true' account, because none of us have unbiased access to our experience. People tend to see yesterday's behaviour through today's lens and so will give different responses according to what has happened subsequently.

Participants are more likely to provide reliable answers to questions if:

- *Efforts are made to aid recall*: some of the devices designed to deal with the problem of candidness – the formulation of neutral questions, and provision of assurances of confidentiality and anonymity – can help the respondent to retrieve information. Ordering questions chronologically in terms of life events aids recall, as does providing well-defined time periods for responses.
- *Privacy is provided for responses*: where feasible, use computer-assisted self-interviewing (CASI, CAPI, and CATI). Where this is not feasible, use other aids

such as show cards, self-completion booklets, and informal confidential voting interview methods.

- *Interviewers adopt a non-judgemental approach*: recruitment and training of interviewers should emphasize the need to maximize comfort and ease on the part of participants. Interviewers should reveal minimal reaction, positive or negative, to what is being reported.
- *Questions are clear, comprehensive, and unambiguous*: general rules about question formulation apply, but in this context it is preferable to ask about *practices* rather than *identities* (for men, for example: 'In your life so far, have you had sex with a man?', as opposed to 'Have you ever had homosexual sex?' (note the impact of the use of 'ever' in the second example, which seems to mark the behaviour off as extraordinary, and so is best avoided).
- *Language used is acceptable*: discomfort with, and misunderstanding of, language will jeopardize willingness to provide accurate responses. Some researchers favour using the participant's vocabulary, others a standardized and neutral terminology, but it is important that both interviewer and interviewee feel comfortable with the language used (see Chapter 11). Beginning with neutral questions, and progressing gradually to more intimate and sensitive ones once rapport has been developed, is an effective strategy for eliciting responses to sensitive data.

The scope of sexual health research

The need to predict and prevent transmission of HIV has provided the impetus to a vast body of sexual behaviour research in recent decades, and has extended research beyond its emphasis on fertility regulation. The complaint that more is known about the sexual behaviour of farmyard animals than that of humans is far less true today than when Alfred Kinsey made it. Yet areas of sexual health remain neglected in terms of empirical study. The investigative gaze could profitably shift away from the current near exclusive emphasis on individual risk factors, for example, towards social contextual determinants of sexual health status. Some population sub-groups, such as men who have sex with men, and some activities, such as transactional sex, are not studied at all in some settings. More attention should be paid to cultural attitudes and social norms that enhance or hinder the implementation of effective preventive interventions and services in this area. More attention is still paid to adverse rather than benign outcomes of sexual behaviour, despite the fact that sexual pleasure and enjoyment may be as important to sexual health status as the number of partners or condom use. A narrow pursuit of data on risk behaviours and risk reduction strategies to the neglect of sexual satisfaction and pleasure may be too limited an approach to do justice to the range of intersections between sexual behaviour and health.

Summary

The need for robust data has in recent decades led to strenuous efforts to overcome the challenges posed by sexual behaviour for scientific enquiry. Innovations in research methods have undoubtedly benefited not only this, but other fields of behavioural enquiry too. The reach of public health investigation into sexual behaviour has also expanded, but there is scope for this to go further still. The need for reliable data on sexual behaviour has provided the impetus for extensive efforts to address the problems of measurement error and bias: to improve the methods used to reach people; to encourage them to take part in research; and to ensure that they are able to give accounts that bear relation to the perceived reality of their lives.

References

Bajos N and Spira A (1992) Analysis of sexual behaviour in France (ACSF). A comparison between two modes of investigation: telephone survey and face-to-face survey, *AIDS*, 6: 315–23.

Cleland J, Boerma JT, Carael M and Weir SS (2004) Monitoring sexual behaviour in general populations: a synthesis of lessons of the past decade, *Sexually Transmitted Infections*, 80(suppl. II): ii1–ii7.

Copas A, Wellings K, Erens B, Mercer CH, McManus S, Fenton KA et al. (2002) The accuracy of reported sensitive sexual behaviour in Britain: exploring the extent of change 1990–2000, *Sexually Transmitted Infections*, 78(1): 26–30.

Fenton KA, Johnson AM, McManus S and Erens B (2001) Measuring sexual behaviour: methodological challenges in survey research, *Sexually Transmitted Infections*, 77: 84–92.

Glynn JR, Kayuni N, Banda E, Parrott F, Floyd S, Francis M et al. (2011) Assessing the validity of sexual behaviour reports in a whole population survey in Rural Malawi, *PLoS One*, 6(7): e22840.

Gregson S, Mushati P, White P, Mlilo M, Mundandi C and Nyamukapa C (2004) Informal confidential voting interview methods and temporal changes in reported sexual risk behaviour for HIV transmission in sub-Saharan Africa, *Sexually Transmitted Infections*, 80(suppl. II): ii36–ii42.

Kinsey AC, Pomeroy WB and Martin CE (1948) *Sexual Behavior in the Human Male*. Philadelphia, PA: WB Saunders.

Kinsey A, Pomeroy W, Martin C and Gebhard P. (1953) *Sexual Behavior in the Human Female*. Philadelphia, PA: WB Saunders.

Marston C and King E (2006) Factors that shape young people's sexual behaviour: a systematic review, *Lancet*, 368(9547): 1581–6.

Masters WH and Johnson VE (1966) *Human Sexual Response*. New York: Bantam Books.

Mitchell K, Wellings K, Elam G, Erens B, Fenton K and Johnson A (2007) How can we facilitate reliable reporting in surveys of sexual behaviour? Evidence from qualitative research, *Culture, Health and Sexuality*, 9(5): 519–31.

Slaymaker E, Bwanika JB, Kasamba I, Lutalo T, Maher D and Todd J (2009) Trends in age at first sex in Uganda: evidence from demographic and health survey data and longitudinal cohorts in Masaka and Rakai, *Sexually Transmitted Infections*, 85(suppl. 1): i12–i19.

Wellings K, Field J, Wadsworth J, Johnson AM, Anderson RM and Bradshaw SA (1990) Sexual lifestyles under scrutiny, *Nature*, 348(6299): 276–9.

Wellings K, Collumbien M, Slaymaker E, Singh S, Hodges Z, Patel D et al. (2006) Sexual behaviour in context: a global perspective, *Lancet*, 368(9548): 1706–28.

Evaluating sexual health interventions

Chris Bonell, Martine Collumbien, Helen Burchett and Meg Wiggins

Overview

In previous chapters, we have described ways of intervening to improve sexual health status and in this chapter we consider how best to evaluate their progress towards that goal. We discuss the importance of evaluation and of setting the right questions in this context. We appraise different evaluation designs and consider how to decide on the most rigorous evaluation, taking account of the research question, the aim and complexity of the intervention, and the context in which it is implemented.

Learning outcomes

After reading this chapter, you will be able to:

- Explain the purpose of evaluation and define evaluation questions
- Select the best design based on the research question
- Understand the challenges of evaluating complex sexual health interventions

Key terms

Formative evaluation: An evaluation aimed at fine-tuning a planned intervention before it is taken to scale for an outcome evaluation.

Outcome evaluation: An evaluation used to establish whether the aim of the intervention has been achieved in terms of intended (and unintended) outcomes.

Process evaluation: An evaluation exploring the way in which an intervention is implemented, delivered, and received.

Transferability: The extent to which an intervention evaluated in one specific setting might be as effective in another defined setting.

Introduction

The purpose of evaluation is to inform the design of effective (and cost-effective) interventions and to prevent harmful or ineffective ones. The impact of an intervention is measured through change in key outcomes (for example, safer sex practices, unintended pregnancies, sexual violence). Before claiming an intervention works, we need to demonstrate that the change in outcome can be attributed to the intervention rather than to factors external to it. Evaluation is also about exploring how the intervention worked or, if it did not, why not. Was everything implemented as planned? Were there unexpected obstacles or harmful side effects? Did intermediate outcomes on the causal pathway between exposure to intervention and outcomes move in the expected direction?

Throughout this book, we have come to understand that sexual health problems have multiple, often interrelated causes at individual, group, and community and even a national level. In Chapter 12, we provided an overview of different approaches to intervention and stressed that a combination of behavioural, biomedical, and structural components are most likely to lead to sustained changes in the health status of individuals and communities. 'Combination' approaches constitute 'complex' interventions, and pose challenges to evaluation (Piot et al., 2008; Hankins and de Zalduondo, 2010). While complexity is not uncommon in public health policy and practice, comprehensive evaluation guidance on complex interventions is both relatively recent (MRC, 2000) and continuously developing. There is increasing recognition that optimal approaches need to be less linear and more flexible, moving beyond the template of clinical trials to include a range of approaches (MRC, 2006; Craig et al., 2008; Hankins and de Zalduondo, 2010).

Even with relatively simple interventions, there is a range of evaluation questions that could be answered and the design of the evaluation research will depend on which of these are thought to need answers: is it about outcomes, processes, causal pathways, all of these?

A key clarifying principle will be what decision will be made based on the results of the evaluation and who will be the main user of the information? Policy-makers are often the ultimate audience for evaluation research and public health professionals need to build the evidence base to inform their decision-making and strengthen the link between good science and sound policy. They need to know what works, for whom, and in what contexts. However, policy-makers do not make decisions based on research evidence alone, and social and political palatability are especially important. For them, accountability will be important to ensure public confidence in how limited resources are deployed.

The evaluation cycle

There are four stages in developing and evaluating interventions (whether they are simple or complex): (1) reviewing the best available evidence and developing theoretical understanding; (2) assessing feasibility of the proposed intervention to examine key uncertainties; (3) evaluating the process of implementation, including ways to course correct; and (4) assessing effectiveness of impact by measuring outcomes. It is important to stress that in practice progressing through these stages is not necessarily linear; early in the assessment of the feasibility or during the process evaluation, observations may lead to changes in the original design of the intervention (MRC, 2006).

Reviewing the evidence and developing theoretical understanding

The more we understand about the determinants of a specific sexual health problem, and the more we know about the context, the better we will be able to design the most appropriate and effective intervention. We may be able to draw on a body of evidence of interventions that have been tried and tested before in diverse settings. Based on existing evidence and theory, we need to develop a theoretical understanding of the intended process of change, to improve planning and ensure that we do not repeat mistakes from the past (MRC, 2006). Detailed causal models of a project implementation pathway (PIP) show how each component is expected to affect the ultimate (or intermediate) outcomes. This clarifies implicit assumptions and helps implementers monitor failing strategies when uncertainties have been flagged (Hankins and de Zalduondo, 2010).

Assessing feasibility

Numerous interventions have been shown to be ineffective in outcome evaluations, due to design problems that could have been solved had the feasibility been assessed (Elford et al., 2000). Feasibility studies, also called 'formative evaluation', often consist of pilot studies to test a range of questions to assess acceptability, compliance, and expected coverage (MRC, 2000). This is especially important with new interventions and those transferred from other contexts.

Activity 16.1

Imagine that a review of existing rigorous outcome evaluations concluded that interventions allowing teenage girls to spend time with toddlers were effective in reducing rates of teenage pregnancy. However, suppose also that all of the programmes in the review were based in the USA. You are about to set up a similar intervention in the UK. What information would you collect in a formative evaluation to assess the feasibility of this? What evaluation questions would you suggest?

Feedback

You might like to implement a pilot study in one area before any wider roll-out. The evaluation could gather qualitative data to explore the experiences of those using the programme, those planning and running the programme, and other key stakeholders, including nurseries, parents, and schools. It could also collect quantitative data on coverage and the acceptability of the programme. The main evaluation questions might be:

• Is it feasible to deliver such a programme in the UK?
• Can the programme reach the target audience (girls at risk of teenage pregnancy)?
• What do the recipients – schools, nurseries, and girls targeted – think of the programme?
• What aspects of the programme need to be changed to maximize the success of the programme in the UK compared with the USA?
• What contextual factors influence feasibility, coverage, and acceptability?

The acceptability of an intervention is important, though not merely as a predictor of likely effectiveness but also in its own terms. Explicit sexual materials may be effective in motivating safer sex practices among the target group of men in London gay bars, but in other public places – whether the waiting room at the GP surgery, a gym or a youth centre – the same materials may be offensive to both the targeted group and the general public.

Evaluating the process of implementation

Documenting *how* the intervention was actually implemented is the main aim of implementation research. Key questions in this context include: Did the actual *process* follow the detailed project implementation pathway (i.e. was it implemented with fidelity)? Was it received as intended? The answers to these need to be documented with enough detail for providers elsewhere to judge whether and how they might reproduce the intervention.

When combined with an *outcome* evaluation, this information increases our understanding of why an intervention was or was not effective and how easy it might be to undertake it in another context.

Activity 16.2

Imagine you are evaluating a mobile family planning clinic in rural sub-Saharan Africa. What questions might your process evaluation ask? Jot down a few ideas.

Feedback

In a process evaluation, we could ask:

- Is the intervention delivered with good fidelity (as intended) or quality (at the standards set for it)?
- Does the intervention achieve good coverage with those it intended to reach?
- Are providers explaining a range of contraceptive options to all clients? Do they accept the needs of unmarried girls or do they tend to discourage them by suggesting that they should not be having sex?
- Is there community opposition from any stakeholders (e.g. traditional healers) who had not been consulted?
- What features of the context appear to act as facilitators for, or barriers against, the feasibility and acceptability of intervention?
- Is evidence from the evaluation likely to be applicable and transferable to a specified other context?
- How does the local context shape the implementation?
- What characteristics of the context help or hinder the intervention?

Process evaluation should aim to examine the intervention from a variety of perspectives using both quantitative and qualitative data. Where a pilot study shows that both managers and nurses in a sexual health clinic believe delivery of their chosen counselling is feasible, is this true in all areas? Does it hold in regions that mainly serve other ethnic groups? Do local providers have the capacity to implement the intervention, and are the authorities supportive? Achieving coverage may depend on the overall comprehensiveness of health systems or on whether providers can reach people in other ways, such as through outreach. Adequate coverage may be more difficult in some sites or among certain sub-populations. Acceptability may also vary between populations. For example, HIV voluntary counselling and testing services that require clients to attend clinics twice (first for testing and then for results) may be acceptable in high-income settings but not low-income settings, where the transport or opportunity costs are too high. These are all matters that a process evaluation can examine with regard to the original evaluation site and in replication studies (Burchett et al., 2011).

In more complex interventions that are designed to be adapted to local circumstances, testing fidelity (the extent to which the programme was implemented as planned in the protocol) may not be clear-cut (Craig et al., 2008). Variability in implementation can be pre-planned or arise through unexpected circumstances. In either case, detailed documentation is needed to explain variation in outcome, underlining the need for rigorous process evaluation (Hawe et al., 2004).

Investigating contextual factors that might influence the delivery of an intervention is an important part of process evaluation. This is also the stage at which we may uncover unintended consequences, whether negative or positive. Major financial investments may accelerate outcomes by driving wider secular changes, while economic downturns or political shocks may lead to smaller than intended effects (Pronyk et al., 2012).

Outcome and process evaluations are not mutually exclusive and are often undertaken together. A process-only evaluation might be sufficient where an intervention, previously found effective in one or more settings, is being replicated in a similar setting (Hargreaves et al., 2010). Since the measurement of impact on health status may require longer evaluation periods, studies to evaluate large-scale HIV prevention programmes need to be designed to allow for the possibility of mid-course corrections based on monitoring intermediate outcomes (Padian et al., 2011).

Outcome evaluation

Many see the question of whether the intervention achieves its aims, that is, 'does it work'?, as being at the heart of the evaluation process. Outcome measures are indicators that are used to assess whether aims have been achieved. Whether or not negative outcomes are prevented or positive outcomes achieved will have important consequences, both for those experiencing the intervention as well as those funding and delivering it. It is therefore important to identify whether interventions are effective, something that cannot be assumed (Bonell et al., 2003). As well as overall outcomes, it may be important to examine the effects an intervention has on specific sub-groups or in particular areas, such as whether it is effective in reducing health inequalities, or in explaining discrepancies between expected and observed outcomes in certain contexts. Evaluations may examine costs as well as outcomes in order to determine an intervention's cost-effectiveness.

Which outcomes?

Interventions need clear aims for outcomes to be identified and measured. Some outcomes may be biological, such as testing of saliva samples for HIV infection; others relate to attitudes or behaviour, and are collected using survey research. Sometimes, especially in the case of the prevention of relatively uncommon outcomes, proxies for the outcome are measured instead of, or in addition to, the outcomes themselves. For example, a proxy for teenage pregnancy might be sexual debut before age 16 (Wellings et al., 2001). Often funders want to see changes in behaviour outcomes or even health impacts, which typically are difficult or slow to achieve.

In complex interventions, outcomes may be at different levels – individual, group, and community level – and not all desired outcomes are necessarily easily measurable. As we saw in Chapter 8, community mobilization programmes targeting sex workers focus on empowering them to change the social environment in which they live. When activities are directed towards enabling people to take action, participation and partnership are *valued processes*, and empowerment of individuals and communities are seen as *valued outcomes* (Nutbeam, 1998). These may be less quantifiable and clearly qualitative studies will be needed to assess how empowerment happens. The documented success of the Sonagachi project (Chapter 8) has come mainly from detailed ethnographic research (Cornish and Ghosh, 2007; Evans and Lambert, 2008; Cornish, 2009). This research warns against the measurement of outcomes dictating the evaluation (and hence the intervention). If we neglect outcomes and processes that are not easily quantifiable, then 'we will measure what is easily evaluable and ignore what is valuable' (Coombes and Thorogood, 2004: 5).

To ensure rigour, evaluators must state what the intended outcomes are *prior to* analysis and report on *all* of these outcomes. This avoids the issue of 'data-dredging', which refers to searching for significant positive outcomes and only reporting these. Instead, all pre-defined outcomes measures, whether positive, negative or showing no change, should be reported. The more measures are considered, the more chance there is that apparently 'significant' statistical results will arise through chance alone. When the intervention is 'simple', it is easier to keep the number of primary or key secondary outcome measures to a minimum. However, for more complex interventions when there is a range of intervention aims, limiting outcomes may not be the best use of data or provide an adequate assessment of the success of interventions (MRC, 2006).

In the next section, we demonstrate that strategies to evaluate the effects of different programmatic interventions cannot be standardized.

Evaluation design

The term 'evaluation design' is used to describe the overall structure and logic of the evaluation (not the research methods used). There are three main types of evaluation design: true experimental, quasi-experimental, and non-experimental designs. The important difference between these designs is the level of inference or attribution that can be made about the intervention causing the outcome. Exposure to an intervention is likely to be associated with other factors that also affect the outcome and thus leads to a selection bias. These factors, called confounders, typically include socio-demographic characteristics such as education and socio-economic status. When they are not controlled for they can cause selection bias.

True experimental designs, such as randomized controlled trials (RCTs), are considered by some to be the only design that can demonstrate causality. In RCTs, units (individuals or clusters, such as schools) are allocated at random to the intervention or control group. This ensures that the intervention and control group are truly comparable and differ only in their exposure to the intervention. Both observed and unobserved confounders are balanced between the study arms and are least affected by selection bias. Randomized controlled trials have the most internal validity.

Randomization may not be possible if policy-makers or providers refuse to allow it, such as if they perceive it to be unethical as there is some confidence that the intervention will be advantageous. Randomized controlled trials are only done when there is uncertainty (equipoise) about the benefit of the intervention. For example, we know condoms work and it would be unethical to test this.

When intervention and control groups cannot be randomized, there is the potential for introducing selection bias, since the exposed and unexposed groups may differ in terms of 'unobserved' confounders. In these *quasi-experimental designs*, a non-randomized control group may be used. This group might comprise individuals who are matched to those receiving the intervention in terms of characteristics thought likely to influence the health outcomes being targeted. With or without matching, evaluators can also measure and adjust for differences that do exist between the intervention and comparison groups. The disadvantage is that they cannot control for unmeasured or imperfectly measured confounders.

Confounding can lead to evaluators underestimating intervention effects if, for example, greater baseline risk among intervention recipients is not sufficiently considered. More commonly, confounding can lead evaluators to overestimate effects, such as when lower baseline risk or a greater propensity to benefit from the intervention is insufficiently considered.

When it is not possible to have a comparison group, such as where policy-makers refuse to deny anyone the intervention, evaluators might consider using a stepped-wedge trial. This staggers the introduction of an intervention to different groups, randomizing the order of receipt rather than whether it received at all. The comparison group is then made up of individuals who have not yet received the intervention. Comparison groups will sometimes be impossible because of legal, bureaucratic or practical barriers, such as when evaluating the effects of legislation, welfare benefits or mass media on sexual health.

Often the same interventions (or similar ones) are already being delivered across an entire area, and there are no naive control groups. This often is the case with HIV prevention programmes. In *observational studies*, internal 'before–after' comparisons may be possible. These are vulnerable to confounding from overall secular trends in the outcome (e.g. overall changes in teenage pregnancy rates over time), maturational trends (e.g. young people becoming more sexually active as they get older), and contemporaneous influential events (e.g. an HIV story in a television drama). The extent to which these undermine an evaluation depends on context: secular trends are less problematic where rates of an outcome among a population are stable and where intervention effects are large and specific. Evidence from before–after studies can be persuasive when assessing new behaviours, such as promoting the use of new forms of contraception.

Activity 16.3

In Chapter 12, we discussed extensively the challenges when designing appropriate HIV interventions. Reflect on the methodological issues you might encounter in evaluating these interventions.

Feedback

> - combination prevention is complex and multi-level;
> - HIV as outcome is rare; no reliable incidence assay
>   ○ large sample sizes/long horizons;
> - inconsistent relationship between HIV and surrogate outcomes (STIs, pregnancy, sexual risk behaviour);
> - proxy of self-reported behaviours often biased;
> - long and multiple causal pathways, with social drivers working indirectly;
> - lack of naive controls
>   ○ measuring marginal effect above existing programmes.
>
> (Padian et al., 2011)

A lack of control group in observational studies does not necessarily mean that they cannot provide rigorous evidence of the impact of an intervention. Indeed, they may be favoured by those primarily focused on evaluation intervention 'in context' – those who are most concerned about structural or social change, and with the interaction between the intervention and the context in which is implemented (Auerbach et al., 2011). HIV prevention relies on human behaviour which has dynamic meanings shaped by societal conditions (Hankins and de Zalduondo, 2010).

Moving to a consensus – cumulative evidence from different designs

What evidence do we have for the pros and cons of using different study designs?

Most success stories have been documented with observational data (Auerbach et al., 2011). Early behaviour change interventions targeting individuals had little impact on sexual risk behaviour despite increases in awareness of risk reduction. Failure was apparent when tested as a single intervention (and effect sizes were too small). At the same time, as we saw in Chapter 12, behaviour change communication was central to all success stories, such as community-based intervention with gay men in the USA and UK, as well as huge declines in HIV incidence in Thailand and Uganda (Coates et al., 2008).

Most RCTs on HIV prevention provide little evidence of effect. Nearly 90% of all HIV intervention trials show 'flat' results, meaning that they could not demonstrate any effect (Padian et al., 2010), including several that tested behavioural interventions. Of the 39 interventions tested, only five showed a positive effect: all of them were biomedical interventions and three were on male circumcision. Importantly, one of the 12 trials on microbicides showed an increase in HIV transmission (due to the abrasive effect of non-oxynol-9), demonstrating how crucial trials are for testing biomedical interventions. However, flat results do *not* mean no effect. Rather, they show that the trial failed to demonstrate an effect because of a variety of issues, including lack of statistical power to detect an effect (due to unexpectedly low incidence in many trials), comparison groups receiving diluted versions of interventions (institutional review boards demand enhanced rather than standard care), and poor adherence (Padian et al., 2010). With this even the most staunch advocates of RCTs had to concede that the pure gold data in the gold standard of evaluation designs needed the strength of steel to forge 'alloys' with data from observational data and other lines of evidence, rather than writing off all interventions with modest levels of effect.

Choosing an evaluation design for your evaluation

While some scientists from biomedical backgrounds will continue to favour experimental designs, there has been increasing interest in non-randomized evaluations of public health interventions (Victora et al., 2004), especially when they are implemented at a large scale. The strength of evidence is expressed either as *adequacy* (change observed but no clear attribution) or *plausibility* (observed changes compared against a non-randomly selected reference group, which could involve a pre and post design or an external control group).

The *public health significance of the* research question determines the evaluation design, which should be as rigorous as possible. The evaluation design needs to be tailored to the research question rather than vice versa; fitting the intervention into the framework of RCTs defeats the purpose of good public health practice (Coates et al., 2008; Thorogood and Coombes, 2010).

Large-scale combination HIV prevention programmes come with their own set of evaluation challenges, and one of them is to identify a valid 'counterfactual' – that is, what would have happened if the intervention had not been implemented. In experimental designs, the counterfactual is 'observed' in the control group. Mathematical modelling may also be used to address the problem of a missing counterfactual.

In general, the more structural the intervention and the more multi-faceted, the less likely it is that we can adopt a probability design. Circumstances under which randomized designs could or should be strongly considered to evaluate structural interventions include: (1) the aim is to assess the efficacy of unproven interventions; (2) interventions can be delivered in a consistent manner across areas; (3) interventions are reasonably 'discrete' and work through pre-specified impact pathways; (4) a large number of units can be randomized; and (5) reasonably unexposed control groups can be maintained throughout the assessment period (Bonell et al., 2006; Victora et al., 2011; Pronyk et al., 2012).

Randomization may not be needed if the effect size of the intervention is predicted to be large and/or the effect immediate. In this case, neither confounding nor secular trends are likely to explain differences in outcomes before and after exposure. On the other hand, when effect sizes are very small, or the effect very long-term, randomized designs may not be feasible (MRC, 2006).

A number of strategies can improve the case for attribution – whether exposure to an intervention has caused the observed changes. Impact pathway mapping involves applying a pre-defined and theoretically grounded impact pathway that systematically maps mechanisms through which an intervention is expected to lead to changes in outcomes. In a complex and multi-component structural intervention, it is important to track indicators at each point in a causal chain. The size and consistency of changes across a range of activities and outcomes also helps enhance the plausibility that observed effects were a result of an intervention, while helping to distinguish between interventions that are inherently faulty (failure of intervention concept or theory), those that were simply badly delivered (implementation failure), and those that were truly ineffective (an intervention that was well conceived, well implemented, but ultimately not effective).

Summary

Evaluation is necessary to examine not only the outcomes but also the process of planning, delivery, and receipt of sexual health interventions. The *public health significance of the* research question should determine the evaluation design, which should be as rigorous as possible. The evaluation itself should not compromise the integrity and effectiveness of a programme.

The optimal design to examine the *effectiveness* of a programme will generally be a randomized controlled trial. This can include a process evaluation to examine the feasibility, coverage, and acceptability of the intervention and how these are influenced by context. Process-only evaluations can be useful in refining new interventions or examining the potential applicability and transferability of established interventions to new settings. In the 'real world' of complex evaluations in which 'background noise' may compromise rigorous experimental approaches, evaluation research must operate with maximum flexibility, a creative mix of methods, and a healthy tolerance for uncertainty.

References

Auerbach JD, Parkhurst JO and Cáceres CF (2011) Addressing social drivers of HIV/AIDS for the long-term response: conceptual and methodological considerations, *Global Public Health*, 6(suppl. 3): S293–S309.

Bonell CP, Bennett R and Oakley A (2003) Sexual health should be subject to experimental evaluation, in J Stephenson, J Imrie and C Bonell (eds.) *Effective Sexual Health Interventions: Issues in Experimental Evaluation*. Oxford: Oxford University Press.

Bonell C, Hargreaves J, Strange V, Pronyk P and Porter J (2006) Should structural interventions be evaluated using RCTs? The case of HIV prevention. *Social Science and Medicine*, 63: 1135–42.

Burchett HED, Umoquit MJ and Dobrow MJ (2011) How do we know when research from one setting can be useful in another? A systematic scoping review of external validity, applicability and transferability frameworks, *Journal of Health Services Research and Policy*, 16: 238–44.

Coates TJ, Richter L and Caceres C (2008) Behavioural strategies to reduce HIV transmission: how to make them work better, *Lancet*, 372(9639): 669–84.

Coombes Y and Thorogood M (2004) Introduction, in M Thorogood and Y Coombes (eds.) *Evaluating Health Promotion: Practice and Methods*. Oxford: Oxford University Press.

Cornish F (2009) Targeting HIV or targeting social change? The role of Indian sex worker collectives in challenging gender relations, in J Boesten and N Poku (eds.) *Gender and HIV/AIDS: Critical Perspectives from the Developing World*. London: Ashgate.

Cornish F and Ghosh R (2007) The necessary contradictions of 'community-led' health promotion: a case study of HIV prevention in an Indian red light district, *Social Science and Medicine*, 64(2): 496–507.

Craig N, Dieppe P, Macintyre S, Michie S, Nazareth I and Petticrew M 2008 Developing and evaluating complex interventions: the new Medical Research Council guidance, *British Medical Journal*, 337: 979–83.

Elford J, Bolding G and Sherr L (2000) Peer education has no significant impact on HIV risk behaviours among gay men in London, *AIDS*, 15(4): 535–8.

Evans C and Lambert H (2008) Implementing community interventions for HIV prevention: insights from project ethnography, *Social Science and Medicine*, 66(2): 467–78.

Hankins CA and de Zalduondo BO (2010) Combination prevention: a deeper understanding of effective HIV prevention, *AIDS*, 24: S70–S80.

Hargreaves J, Hatcher A, Strange V, Phetla G, Busza J, Euripidou R et al. (2010) Group-microfinance and health promotion among the poor: six-year process evaluation of the Intervention with Microfinance for AIDS and Gender Equity (IMAGE) in rural South Africa, *Health Education Research*, 25(1): 27–40.

Hawe P, Shiell A and Riley T (2004) Complex interventions: how 'out of control' can a randomised trial be?, *British Medical Journal*, 328: 1561–3.

Medical Research Council (MRC) (2000) *A Framework for Development and Evaluation of RCTs for Complex Interventions to Improve Health*. London: MRC.

Medical Research Council (MRC) (2006) *Developing and Evaluating Complex Interventions: New Guidance*. London: UK-MRC.

Nutbeam D (1998) Evaluating health promotion – progress, problems and solutions, *Health Promotion International*, 13(1): 27–44.

Padian NS, McCoy SI, Balkus J and Wasserheit JN (2010) Challenges in HIV prevention research: weighing the gold in the gold standard, *AIDS*, 24(9): 621–35.

Padian N, McCoy SI, Manian S, Wilson D, Schwartlander B & Bertozzi S (2011) Evaluation of combination HIV prevention programs: essential issues, *Journal of Acquired Immune Deficiency Syndrome*, 53: e23–e28.

Piot P, Bartos M, Larson H, Zewdie D and Mane P (2008) Coming to terms with complexity: a call to action for HIV prevention, *Lancet*, 372(9641): 845–59.

Pronyk P, Schaefer J, Somers M and Heise L (2012) Evaluating structural interventions in public health: challenges, options and global best-practice, in M Sommer and R Parker (eds.) *Structural Approaches in Public Health*. London: Routledge.

Thorogood M and Coombes Y (eds.) (2010) *Evaluating Health Promotion, Practice and Methods*. Oxford: Oxford University Press.

Victora C, Habicht JP and Bryce J (2004) Evidence-based public health: moving beyond randomized trials, *American Journal of Public Health*, 94(3): 400–5.

Victora CG, Black RE, Boerma JT and Bryce J. (2011) Measuring impact in the Millennium Development Goal era and beyond: a new approach to large-scale effectiveness evaluations, *Lancet*, 377: 85–95.

Wellings K, Nanchahal K, MacDowall W, McManus S, Erens B, Mercer C et al. (2001) Sexual behaviour in Britain: early heterosexual experience, *Lancet*, 358: 1843–9.

Further reading

Bonell C, Hargreaves J, Cousens S, Ross D, Hayes R, Petticrew M et al. (2011) Alternatives to randomisation in the evaluation of public-health interventions: design challenges and solutions, *Journal of Epidemiology and Community Health*, 65: 576–81.

Craig N, Dieppe P, Macintyre S, Michie S, Nazareth I and Petticrew M (2008) Developing and evaluating complex interventions: the new Medical Research Council guidance, *British Medical Journal*, 337: a1655.

Medical Research Council (MRC) (2006) *Developing and Evaluating Complex Interventions: New Guidance*. London: UK-MRC.

Thorogood M and Coombes Y (eds.) (2010) *Evaluating Health Promotion, Practice and Methods*. Oxford: Oxford University Press.

Index

Page numbers in *italics* refer to figures and tables.

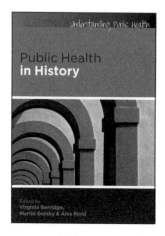

PUBLIC HEALTH IN HISTORY

Virginia Berridge, Martin Gorsky
and Alex Mold

9780335242641 (Paperback)
2011

eBook also available

This fascinating book offers a wide ranging exploration of the history of
public health and the development of health services over the past two
centuries. The book surveys the rise and redefinition of public health
since the sanitary revolution of the mid-nineteenth century, assessing
the reforms in the post World War II years and the coming of welfare
states.

Written by experts from the London School of Hygiene and Tropical
Medicine, this is the definitive history of public health.

Key features:

- Case studies on malaria, sexual health, alcohol and substance
  abuse
- A comparative examination of why healthcare has taken such
  different trajectories in different countries
- Exercises enabling readers to easily interact with and critically
  assess historical source material

www.openup.co.uk

OPEN UNIVERSITY PRESS
McGraw · Hill Education

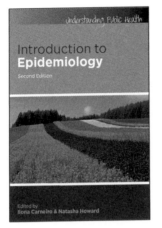

INTRODUCTION TO EPIDEMIOLOGY
Second Edition

Ilona Carneiro and Natasha Howard

9780335244614 (Paperback)
September 2011

eBook also available

This popular book introduces the principles, methods and application
of epidemiology for improving health and survival. It assists readers in
applying basic epidemiological methods to measure health outcomes,
identifying risk factors for a negative outcome, and evaluating health
interventions and health services.

The book also helps to distinguish between strong and poor
epidemiological evidence; an ability that is fundamental to promoting
evidence-based health care.

Key features:

- A broad range of examples and activities covering a range of
  contemporary health issues including obesity, mental health and
  cervical cancer
- New chapter on study design and data handling
- Updated and additional exercises for self-testing

OPEN UNIVERSITY PRESS
McGraw - Hill Education

www.openup.co.uk

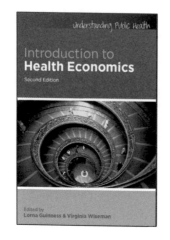

INTRODUCTION TO HEALTH ECONOMICS
Second Edition

Lorna Guinness and Virginia Wiseman

9780335243563 (Paperback)
September 2011

eBook also available

This practical text offers the ideal introduction to the economic techniques used in public health and is accessible enough for those who have no or limited knowledge of economics. Written in a user-friendly manner, the book covers key economic principles, such as supply and demand, healthcare markets, healthcare finance and economic evaluation.

Key features:

- Extensive use of global examples from low, middle and high income countries, real case studies and exercises to facilitate the understanding of economic concepts
- A greater emphasis on the practical application of economic theories and concepts to the formulation of health policy
- New chapters on macroeconomics, globalization and health and provider payments

www.openup.co.uk

OPEN UNIVERSITY PRESS
McGraw · Hill Education

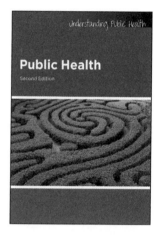

ISSUES IN PUBLIC HEALTH
Second Edition

Fiona Sim and Martin McKee

9780335244225 (Paperback)
September 2011

eBook also available

What is public health and why is it important? By looking at the foundations of public health, its historical evolution, the themes that underpin public health and the increasing importance of globalization, this book provides thorough answers to these two important questions.

Written by experts in the field, the book discusses the core issues of modern public health, such as tackling vested interests head on, empowering people so they can make healthy decisions, and recognising the political nature of the issues. The new edition has been updated to identify good modern public health practice, evolving from evidence

Key features:

- New chapters on the expanding role of public health, covering the issues of sustainability and climate change, human rights, genetics and armed conflict
- Examination of the impact of globalization on higher and lower income countries
- Expanded UK and International examples

www.openup.co.uk

OPEN UNIVERSITY PRESS
McGraw - Hill Education

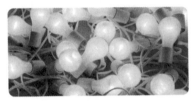 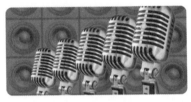
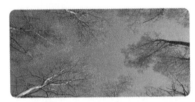 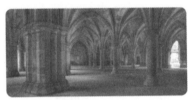
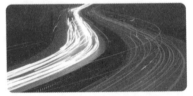 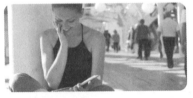
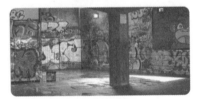